Published 2021 by Dynamite Books

www.dynamitebookspublishing.com

ASIN: 9798790106514

Cover design by Dynamite Books.

First printing, December 2021.

D1710243

Dynamite Books, LLC

2

CONTENTS

INTRODUCTION

Chapter 1 What Can Keto Do for You?

Chapter 2 Frequently Asked Questions About Keto

Chapter 3 What the Heck Am I Supposed to Eat, Mayo?

Chapter 4 Tracking and Getting Results: Exactly How Many Carbs Can I Eat and Still Lose Weight?

Chapter 5 Getting Through the First Three Weeks, AKA "Keto Hell"

Chapter 6 How to Tell Whether You're in Ketosis

Chapter 7 Easy Beverages That Legitimately Taste Good

Chapter 8 Easy Breakfasts That Legitimately Taste Good

Chapter 9 Easy Lunches That Legitimately Taste Good

Chapter 10 Easy Dinners That Legitimately Taste Good

Chapter 11 Easy Snacks That Legitimately Taste Good

Chapter 12 Easy Desserts That Legitimately Taste Good

Chapter 13 Eating Out on Keto

Chapter 14 Two-Week Meal Plan and Shopping List

Chapter 15 Cheating on Keto the Smart Way

Chapter 16 Keto and Exercise

Chapter 17 What You Need to Know About Intermittent Fasting and Keto

Chapter 18 Pep Talk: Do NOT Read Until You Need It

A Note From the Author

INTRODUCTION

Who is this book for? Not you, gym rat with 12 percent body fat who talks like they're the first human being to discover physical fitness. If the words "macros" and "feeding window" are part of your vocabulary, you can move right along. There are a ton of books out there for you written by other gym-bros who can help you achieve your dream of 10 percent body fat and ultimate HIIT workouts.

This one is for the average Jill (or Joe). The ones who really want to try keto but are in a love affair with tacos. The ones with two kids who are definitely going to eat mac and cheese sloppily in front of you on your first day of eating keto.

This book is for those of you who aren't willing to give up tacos or pizza but still want to lose the extra 15 pounds or 40 that have been hanging around since they had that baby (who is now ten). The folks who keep hearing about keto but think it sounds like a drag. Or who tried keto for two days and gave up after consuming large quantities of bacon and cheese.

I'm here to tell you what works, without any nonsense. No recipes that sound good but taste gross. No big promises full of hot air. No lingo or health jargon. No impossible asks.

Just real life, down-to-earth advice. And real (yummy) recipes to go with that advice.

The advice I'm sharing in this book is the same advice I've shared with my friends when they ask how I lost thirty pounds. It's the same advice they share with their friends. It's not a blog post full of affiliate links to get you to buy the ingredients for keto donuts that taste like a high-fiber chemical toilet. It's just what works. And what tastes good, so you can actually still enjoy your life while reaching your goals.

This book is for you, especially if you're feeling a little unsure. Especially if you don't know where to start. Especially if you wonder if you can hack it given that you don't know what a "net carb" is.

Because if I can do it, you can do it. And I'm going to tell you how.

Real Talk: The 4-1-1 on Keto

I've learned that you can read fifty blog posts or articles about keto and come out the other side more confused than you went in. Between affiliate links, click bait, the pressure to get more views, and SEO, the real talk—the real stuff you need to know to get started with keto—is spread in little pockets throughout the Internet. The real nuggets of gold, the information that makes you think, "Okay, I get it now," isn't easy to find in one place. Because that wouldn't be a very successful blog.

That's a big part of the reason I wrote this book. Because here's what I would tell you if the two of us were sitting on my couch and you asked me, "Okay, but really, what's the REAL deal with keto?"

The following questions are the biggest mental hurdles and concerns I had—and the biggest questions most people have—before they decide whether keto is worth trying. There's a lot of misinformation and half-true information and confusing information out there. Especially if you're trying to learn about keto from the man-blogger who runs ultra-marathons (this demographic is weirdly over-represented when it comes to resources about keto).

So, let's start here. Because knowing WHY keto works and HOW keto works is actually really important. Like many of you, I grew up in the "fat is bad" era, where we ate low-fat everything. Fat was the enemy. Fat made you fat. And when we got fat anyway, we doubled down. All this is to say that the idea of eating fat to lose fat sounded like the literal definition of crazy when I first heard about keto.

It. Did. Not. Compute.

Who were these idiots telling me to eat fat? My first thought was that scene in *Mean Girls* where Cady convinces Regina, queen of the mean girls, to eat tons of butter for revenge. Who were these people that wanted me to become fat? *Mean.*

Fortunately, I had a girlfriend—Allie—who also happens to be a nutritionist, who set me straight on a few key points. I was skeptical at first. The fear of fat was a big part of me. But Allie is a badass, and everything she said was easy to verify.

In fact, Allie asked me to join her team of researchers for a new keto supplement she was developing (don't worry, I'm not here to sell you that supplement. You don't need it to succeed at keto, and Allie has moved on to a different project anyway). In other words, I had the opportunity to really dig into the claims, research, and evidence for the keto diet. And what I found was surprising in a very good way.

Here's what you need to know:

What Keto Is—and Isn't

There are a LOT of weird, partially true rumors flying around about keto. Which makes sense. The diet totally subverts the way a lot of us think about food at a core level. So, at a very basic level, here is what keto is: A way of eating that replaces the bulk of simple sugars and carbs (one energy source your body can use to fuel you) with fats and proteins (another energy source your body can use to fuel you).

So, is keto "radical"? Yeah, kind of. But in a good way. Because keto literally changes the way your body turns food into energy. See, we've really only been relying on processed carbs (and even a lot of complex, unprocessed carbs) for the last couple of centuries. Before that, before modern society, we relied primarily on fat and protein for the bulk of our fuel.

Ever watch the show Alone? (If you haven't, it's a hardcore survivor show where they drop people in the middle of the wilderness and see how long they can hack it.) What you notice very quickly is that fat and protein become the name of the game. Berries and roughage are vital for micronutrients and fiber, but a "low-fat diet" is not conducive to survival. Those people who eat a low-fat diet go home. The ones who win the show find sources of fat and protein. That's how the majority of our ancestors lived. Yeah, there were grains (high fiber, nothing-like-the-bread-in-your-pantry grains) and vegetables (which fit into a keto diet as well).

The key thing to remember here is that fat and protein were our staples way, way before processed bread and carbs were our staples. And the truth is, our bodies don't evolve THAT fast. Study after study shows us that processed carbs and refined sugar wreak havoc on our systems and contribute to a ton of diseases.

So, keto isn't new. It's just radical when compared with how we've shifted to embrace convenience and processing as part of modern society —often at the expense of our health in the long term.

13

Why Do We Need Keto, Anyway?

I'm going to get a little sciencey on you. Stay with me. Because here's the analogy that helped it finally click for me:

Your body is like a hybrid car. Except instead of running on either gas or electricity, it can run on either fat (in the form of fat molecules + ketones produced in your liver) or sugar (in the form of glycogen molecules).

Your body's primary goal is to be efficient. Which means that, if given the choice, it will opt for simple sugars every time. Why? The reason lies in the fact that your body's systems are pretty ancient. They evolved for millions of years, during which fat and protein were the dominant sources of energy. If you found sweet berries, you loaded up. (And stored any excess sugar as fat for leaner times!) Your brain also rewarded you with a dopamine rush for providing that sugar. Because your brain is a glucose hog. It needs glycogen to work properly. And when your brain didn't have berries as a quick jolt of sugar, it created the glycogen it needed from protein through a process called "gluconeogenesis." And gluconeogenesis isn't nearly as simple as a sugar rush (and also harder to say).

All that worked out fine. Until we hit the industrial revolution and mass production of packaged, processed food. What is processing, exactly? Most of the time, it means altering a food in such a way that it removes a lot of the fiber. E.g., berries have a ton of fiber. Berry syrup doesn't. Sugar cane has a lot of fiber. Refined sugar doesn't. Wheat is full of fiber. Refined, processed flour isn't.

All this means that in today's world, our "sugar" sources are a lot less nutritious than berries most of the time. We have now refined basically everything, from our bread to our treats to our side dishes to our main dishes to our drinks.

Now we're getting to the point. Ready? Here it is: Unfortunately, your brain still thinks that sugar is a rare treat. Even when it's so abundant that we can (and often do) consume it for every meal.

And because your body doesn't have the ability to evolve nearly fast enough to keep up with this shift in food consumption, we don't fare so well on our current diet.

Because when your brain is offered the choice between a simple energy source (like carbohydrates and simple sugars) and a more complex energy source (fats and proteins), your body will default to the quickest, simplest source of energy. Despite the fact that the new simple sugar source isn't good fuel at the end of the day. It's very hard to refuse simple sugar. Because over millions of years, your body associated that tantalizing simple sugar with quick energy, instant brain energy, and increased odds of survival.

Enter keto. You see where we're going, right?

How Keto Works

Keto is a reset that most of us desperately need. And not just because our pants don't fit. (Honestly, this was my biggest motivation for losing weight at first. PANTS ARE EXPENSIVE.)

By shifting to a diet high in healthy fats and adequate protein for gluconeogenesis (as well as some non-processed sources of carbs that have their fiber still intact!) you can do more than lose weight. You can improve a whole slew of side effects that come from a lifetime of relying on processed carbs and sugar—with a body that isn't meant to run on processed carbs and sugar.

If you're like me, you "tried" keto before you actually DID keto (and by that I mean you tried to avoid carbs for a few days, felt HORRIBLE, then went out for pizza).

I want us to get on the same page about that right here. Keto *works*. And keto is a sustainable, healthy diet that realigns your energy consumption with your body's digestive system. But it doesn't feel good at first. In fact, it feels bad for the first few days (the first few days are the hardest), with withdrawals from refined sugar extending into the first three weeks of your adjustment to this diet.

"Why do I feel so bad?" you ask, smugly, "if this is the way my body is SUPPOSED to process energy?"

Okay, smartass (...I asked the same question). It takes a little while for a body that's been heavily reliant on processed and refined carbohydrates to adjust to eating fats and proteins again as the bulk of your diet. EVEN though it's good for you. EVEN though that's the way humans were meant to process energy.

Think of it this way: If you're very out of shape and haven't done any kind of physical activity, it takes a while to be able to walk a mile without feeling terrible, right? If you tried to run a mile after a year of lying in bed, you might think you were going to die. You might think that running a mile was bad for you. You might think that running a mile was hurting you. But if you persist and understand the value of exercise, you'll find that after a period of time you feel way better than you ever did lying in bed.

Living in a state where walking a mile is doable is the ideal. Just like living in a state where your body processes fats and proteins for fuel (instead of sugar nonstop) is the ideal way your body was made to process fuel. That's keto at its very simplest definition.

So … What Happens When I Start Eating Fat? Won't I GET Fat?

Honey, you're already fat. Just kidding, I can't see you and I have no idea what you look like. But that's what I told myself when I decided to conquer my fears about fat and try the keto diet for real. I was already fat. I was already in a place where my pants didn't fit. I was willing to try eating fat. And honestly, it sounded kind of fun to be able to eat butter when I wanted it instead of restricting that. I love butter. Who doesn't love butter?

Anyway, the short answer is no, eating fat won't make you fat. Your body stores excess SUGAR as fat. AKA, burger buns, ice cream, white bread, and soda.

When you stop eating so much simple sugar and simple carbs (aka glucose) and replace that fuel with fat, here's what happens in your body. Your glycogen levels (fuel) that your body stores will go down. And when that happens, your liver will start producing a kind of molecule called "ketones." Ketones exist for the purpose of turning stored fat and consumed fat into energy your body and brain can use for fuel.

That process of turning fat into energy is what we call "ketosis."

You'll notice that earlier I mentioned that a keto diet revolves around fat, adequate protein, and some non-refined carbs. Why just "adequate" protein, instead of high protein? Your body needs protein. Protein isn't a bad dude. In fact, protein is brain and muscle fuel.

(Remember how your body can turn protein into glycogen for your brain fuel?) If you consume a ton of protein (more than you need) however, your body is gonna zap that stuff into glycogen and store it as fat. And we're not here for that.

I'm Gonna Say It … MACROS (Say that like "Mufasa")

Ugh. I hate the word "macros." Any time a person comes at me saying the word "macros" I want to die. Because it's usually a dude wearing a tight black tank top holding a water bottle full of brown sludge.

But the word has to be said. I'm really sorry about that. I feel the pain too.

Here's the deal: "Macros" in the keto sense is just a way to say "percentages of food type that you eat." And in a keto diet, you generally want to arrange your intake like this:

- About 70 percent fats
- About 15-25 percent protein
- About 5-10 percent non-processed carbs (30-50 grams of net carbs. Usually you'll want to stay under 50 grams of net carbs. Don't worry, I'll explain what "net carb" means in a bit. SO MUCH LINGO.)

That's all "macros" means. It helps to track your food intake with an app (there are a bunch of free ones, Carb Manager is my favorite) while you're getting started. It's not always super intuitive which foods are very high in carbohydrates. But the good news is that most people have success counting CARBS rather than CALORIES. In other words, if you stay under your daily allotment of net carbs, you can eat what you need until you feel full. For those of us who have tried a lot of diets that mostly revolved around feeling hungry, this is a breath of fresh air.

I feel like my body is far less stressed and willing to let go of fat on a keto diet in part because I'm genuinely not hungry all the time and in a state of panic about when I can eat next. If I feel hungry, I eat something. I just make sure I'm not snacking on processed carbs.

CHAPTER 1
What Can Keto Do for You?

(You should say that headline in a salesy, slogan voice. It's fun.)

There are basically three main reasons you may want to eat keto: weight loss, health issues, and exercise performance. The vast majority of you are probably looking for a way to lose weight. That's the biggest reason that the diet has been in the spotlight in recent years.

BUT did you know that the keto diet was actually created decades ago as a way to (very successfully) treat childhood epilepsy? How cool is that? The point in me telling you this is that keto actually has WAY more applications than weight loss. So, I want to do a quick dive into the other unsung benefits of keto as well, in case they open anyone's eyes to possible perks that go beyond fitting into your pants. There are OODLES of studies that back these claims up, by the way. Keto is not so much a fad as it is a very cool, very interesting way of shifting energy consumption that has a ton of far-reaching effects.

So, here's the scoop on what keto can do. Since this book focuses mainly on keto as a weight loss option, I'm going to focus this section on the other two benefits of a keto diet: health issues and exercise performance.

Health Benefits

Like I keep saying, keto fundamentally changes the way your body uses energy. That's a big deal. The period of time during which your body is adapting back to using mainly fat for energy is a period in which your body is hard at work. Your mitochondria, the most basic energy-production system in your cells, are changing on a fundamental level. You're essentially creating new energy processing plants in the mitochondria throughout your millions of cells.

Gut and Hormone Health

Keto totally transforms your gut. See, your gut (like the rest of your body) wasn't exactly made for processing refined carbs and sugar. In fact, refined carbs and sugar wreak havoc on your gut. The microbes that should be flourishing there, converting your food into energy, and creating short-chain fatty acids that help your body produce hormones properly, thrive on a high-fiber, low-sugar diet.

A low-carb diet is the ideal environment for good bacteria to flourish in your gut and help you digest your food properly. (Not to mention produce hormones properly. Did you know that the bulk of your serotonin and dopamine are produced in your GUT? That's reason enough to go keto right there.)

Mental Clarity

When your body is reliant on sugar for energy, that means you need a relatively steady stream of food intake to avoid a sudden crash. That's what we call "hangry," folks. When your body gets low on carbs, it sends out an alert system in the form of hunger pangs. If you don't listen, your body amps things up to basically say, "HEY. Where's the FOOD? Our glycogen (or sugar) stores are running low!"

When you rewire your body to rely on fats and proteins instead of sugar, your body is primed to dip into your fat stores for energy WITHOUT sounding the alarm with hangry vibes. Your mental clarity and mood in general don't ebb and flow nearly as much, depending on whether you've eaten a bagel recently.

Improved Inflammation

Ketones (the particular kind of molecule produced in your liver that turn fat into energy) are pretty cool all by themselves. Ketones have actually been shown to block NLRP3 inflammasomes, which studies have consistently connected with insulin resistance, inflammation, and even obesity. Some folks with inflammatory or autoimmune conditions like Rheumatoid Arthritis have had a lot of success improving their symptoms with keto.

A Buttload of Medical Conditions

Remember how I told you that keto was developed to treat epilepsy? Well, that's not all. Here's a few of the biggest mainstream studies and health conditions that are linked to improvement with keto:

Epilepsy

Epilepsy treatment is the origin story of the keto diet. There are TONS of studies documenting keto's effectiveness in managing and treating epilepsy. Many people are able to reach full remission, and those who don't have SIGNIFICANTLY fewer seizures or are sometimes able to stop taking other medicines (which can have rough side effects).

Diabetes

Keto and diabetes patients are a match made in heaven. In studies, keto shows a ton of promise for treating, managing, and even preventing type 2 diabetes. Shifting to heart-healthy fats for energy instead of carbs means that blood glucose levels don't rise and fall so erratically. Keto can also improve symptoms and facilitate healthy weight loss. If you have type 2 diabetes, it's important that you get medical help while shifting to a keto diet. There's a lot of factors at play here, and I want you to stay SAFE most of all.

Migraines

Migraines are commonly triggered by the rise and fall in blood sugar levels. That's why keto, which gets rid of those erratic jumps, is fantastic for migraines. Lots of people find that by switching to a keto diet, they knock out their migraines.

Cancer

Did you know that cancer cells rely on sugar to survive? Crazy, right? So it's not a huge surprise that pilot studies show promising results in treating cancer with keto. Cancer cells are severely compromised in a low-insulin, low-glycogen environment.

Crohn's

Inflammation in the gut is the root of Crohn's disease. That's the reason a LOT of people have found relief from symptoms through keto. As gut health improves and inflammation goes down in the gut, symptoms often subside.

PCOS (Polycystic Ovary Syndrome)

PCOS is a condition that causes infertility, obesity, acne, and excess body hair. Several studies have shown a ton of promise with keto and PCOS. Even MILDLY reducing carb intake can make a big difference for symptoms. And keto itself can even reverse PCOS in some cases.

Alzheimer's

Yep, even Alzheimer's responds to keto. A number of scientists think the diet could be key to preventing or improving Alzheimer's disease. Insulin resistance commonly goes hand in hand with Alzheimer's, crippling cognitive function. We're just beginning to understand all the implications of low-carb living on memory and cognition, but the initial findings are pretty amazing.

Parkinson's

Keto also shows promise for Parkinson's in preventing and treating the disease, for similar reasons it seems to work for Alzheimer's. The keto diet has a ton of potential for neuroprotection in general.

Exercise and Gym Stuff

If you can't tell, I don't love exercising. Don't get me wrong, I know it's good for me. And I do it. Mostly when it's disguised as a walk with my kids and husband, or yard work motivated by fear that my neighbors will judge me.

I have a lot of feelings about the fact that the keto diet is really good for physical endurance. But you might not! So let's talk about that. Keto improves physical endurance the same way it improves mental clarity. When you rely on carbohydrates for energy, you ride a rollercoaster of energy supply. But when you use ketones and fat (consumed AND stored) for energy, you can access that energy in a more stable, consistent way. That means you can access energy more easily any time you need it. So, for anyone who just loves P90X (WHY), you're gonna find a whole new lease on life.

Whether you weight train, run, walk, you name it—keto has been proven to increase endurance significantly. That means you can exercise longer, more intensely, and without feeling like crap. Yay! (We'll have a whole chapter on keto and exercise later, never fear.)

CHAPTER 2
Frequently Asked Questions About Keto

I'll bet you have a few questions right about now. And I have a few answers based on my own experience and a whole lot of research during the time I spent working for a keto supplements company (again, I don't work there anymore, and I'm not trying to sell you anything).

You can skim these questions at your leisure or come back to this section when you need it. It'll be here for you.

How is Keto Different from Atkins?

Keto and Atkins have some similarities. This is true. In fact, they have a lot of similarities. When you tell people that you are doing keto, you're gonna get a lot of confused looks and "Uh, you mean Atkins?" responses.

But keto isn't Atkins. There are a few pretty big differences that actually help explain why keto is so effective.

First, similarities: Both keto and Atkins are focused on low-carb living with the goal of losing weight and improving overall health. However, Atkins is more focused on higher protein and moderate fat, while keto focuses on higher fat and moderate protein.

Now, let's look at differences:

Atkins

Atkins has four phases, and phase one starts out like a keto diet. Basically, you stay below twenty grams of carbs for two weeks. Not insignificantly, this is the phase where you lose the most weight. In phases two and three, you gradually add in more carbs (complex carbs, nature's carbs!) like veggies, fruits, and grains. Phase four is basically an experimental phase, where you see how much variety (and complex

25

carbs) you can add back into your diet while maintaining your weight loss and health goals. You can go back to phases one, two, or three if you need to lose more weight or don't see the health benefits you want.

Since you don't spend a lot of time in the "keto" phase of the Atkins diet, most Atkins dieters don't actually become fat adapted. (E.g., where the body really embraces using fat for fuel. It's more of a shock to the system and then a reintroduction of certain carbs.)

Keto

Most people will tell you there's only one phase of the keto diet: the one where you reduce your carb intake to 30-50 grams per day, on a consistent basis. There IS going to be some experimentation to learn where your body does best. Some people can easily remain in ketosis on 50 grams of net carbs. (I know, I keep saying that phrase. We'll get to net carbs.) But other people find that closer to 20 or 30 grams of carbs per day is the magic number for their weight loss and health goals. Regardless of your magic carb number, the goal of keto is to become FAT ADAPTED. Not to flirt with keto for a couple of weeks. To get into a new relationship with food and your body. This process of fat adaption can take anywhere from a few weeks to a few months. And here's the great news. When you become fat adapted, you won't feel that "shock to your system" anymore where you miss refined carbs like crazy. I know that sounds impossible, but I swear it's true. Once you adapt, eating keto is pretty darn enjoyable, intuitive, and easy.

Like I said earlier, keto focuses on MACROS (MUFASA). So, around 70% fat, 20% protein, 5% carbs. Not phases. Why not "the more protein the better"? Because your body can convert protein into glycogen (aka, sugar).

Because of the focus on fat adaption, the health benefits that go hand in hand with keto are more impressive than Atkins. There's documented evidence for weight loss, improved insulin sensitivity, and a whole slew of documented medical benefits that we mentioned earlier.

Keto isn't "better" than Atkins, per se. It depends on your goals. If you're serious about weight loss and health benefits, keto is probably your gal. But some people find that the increased food variety Atkins offers (along with some health benefits!) is just more doable. I get it. I love food.

I personally like to incorporate a bit of Atkins into my diet for the long-term. I spent several months in the keto phase (to meet my weight loss goals and truly adapt to using fat). But after that, I incorporated some of the carbier whole food fruits and veggies I missed into my diet in moderation (like carrots, for instance). This helps me maintain metabolic flexibility. (E.g., my body can use fat or complex carbohydrates for energy easily and keeps my diet sustainable.) I don't try to add in a bunch of white bread or donuts. Because that stuff was never good for me, and I don't crave it anymore. But peaches? Oh yeah. Micronutrients and metabolic flexibility taste great. I know there are some diehard keto fatheads out there (I see you, 10 percent body fat bro) who are screaming into the void right now. But keep screaming, man. I'm gonna eat the peach.

The reason I bring up Atkins at all (aside from the fact that people WILL confuse keto and Atkins constantly) is the idea of flexibility. I'm not here to evangelize keto. I'm here to explain it in a way that makes sense and helps you decide if it's a good fit for you. And I'm also here to tell you that you don't get any life points for being THE MOST KETO EVER. You get life points for doing what works, feeling good, and enjoying the food you eat while fueling and loving your body. And any shift away from heavy reliance on refined, processed carbs and sugar is a good thing. Because it might taste good at the moment, but there's really no doubt that this stuff is hurting our bodies.

Basically, take what works from good information sources, make sustainable choices, and don't be a jerk about what other people decide to do. And don't fight me about the peach.

Counting Carbs: AKA, What the HECK Is a Net Carb?

Yay! Net carbs! Isn't that a ridiculous-sounding name? I hate diet lingo. But you're gonna hear this particular phrase all the time, and I don't want to confuse you. So NET CARB. GET THOSE NET CARBS IN YOUR MACROS (Gross).

Net carbs are the result of finding the carb count of a particular food, then subtracting fiber and sugar alcohols. Because fiber and sugar alcohols don't count.

Weird, right? Let me explain a little.

Your body can't digest certain types of carbs (fiber and sugar alcohols). These carbs don't count. So you subtract them out and worry about your NET carbs (the carbs left over after subtracting out fiber and sugar alcohol). You only need to count your net carbs when you're doing keto. Essentially, if you eat a piece of bread that contains 12 grams of carbs and 12 grams of fiber, you get a zero net carb count. (There is such a low-carb bread, and I will tell you about it later. It's magic.)

Why? Fiber goes straight to your colon. It's good stuff. It helps you poop normally. AND it doesn't count toward your daily carb load or raise your blood sugar. Fiber is the hero we all need, especially on a keto diet. Some keto purists refuse to count net carbs. Which, in my experience, is a pretty difficult approach to keto. Sugar alcohols on the other hand, are a trickier matter. Sugar alcohols briefly enter the bloodstream, then go straight into your urine. They CAN affect your blood sugar (although MUCH less than real sugar) and are partly absorbed in the small intestines. And if you eat too many sugar alcohols, you might get really intense diarrhea.

The takeaway? Fiber is generally your friend. (although if you eat like, 10 times your daily recommended value, you might feel gross. As with basically anything.) Sugar alcohols can make your diet more varied and enjoyable but use them more sparingly. Neither count toward your "net carbs" for the day.

And no, you can't eat a bunch of fiber in one food and a bunch of sugar in another food and cancel the transaction. That won't fly. We're talking about food on a molecular level here!

Do I Need to Count Calories on Keto?

Here's the good news: Most people do NOT need to count calories on a ketogenic diet. Why? Because as you become fat adapted and stop relying on carbs, your body becomes WAY better at telling you when it's full.

How is that possible? Well, did you know that your body has hormonal "satiety" triggers that fire when you consume protein, fiber, and fat? Yes indeed. But your body does NOT have satiety triggers for isolated carbohydrates. In nature, carbohydrates come with fiber. They're a package deal. It's really not possible to find carbs without fiber in any quantity. But when we refine and process nature's carbs (and remove the fiber), we take away the triggers that tell your body it's full. Ever hear a kid tell you that they are "full of dinner but have room for dessert"? Have you ever thought that yourself? That's because your body has no built-in trigger to tell you when it's full of processed carbs. Meaning, we tend to overeat these foods until our stomach itself is literally full to the point of pain. Far beyond the point of being nutritionally satisfied and full to the point of satisfying hunger.

This is fantastic news for keto dieters. You don't need to obsess over calories. You just need to keep an eye on your net carbs. It's extremely difficult to overeat on fat, protein, and whole food carbohydrates (like berries and veggies). You will feel full before you overeat. For those of you who have tried a lot of diets, this might sound impossible. But give it a try. This is actually one of the things I love best about a keto diet. I hate being hungry. I hate counting calories. I feel deprived and stressed out, and it's hard to stick to a diet when you feel that way.

With keto, I eat whenever I am hungry. If I don't have carbs left for the day, I eat a zero-carb snack (there are lots of good options).

Pretty awesome, right? If you don't believe me, go ahead and track your intake of food. Use an app that's designed to count carbs first and calories second (e.g., Carb Manager). Pay attention to your carbs. And at the end of the day, look at your calories. Don't go hungry. But stick to your carb count. You'll be surprised by how few calories you're consuming compared to your normal intake, while feeling full!

How Much Weight Can I Lose and How Quickly?

How much weight you can lose with the keto diet depends mostly on how quickly your body adapts to the diet and how well you follow it. If you're "cheating" every other day, your body won't switch over to using fat as a fuel source very effectively. Instead, it'll continue to crave and seek carbs as your primary fuel source. You might lose some weight, but you won't make the shift from using carbs to using fat as fuel in any real way.

I can't tell you how many people who have "tried" keto and then reported they lost zero weight. But on further inspection, they were eating WAY more than the carbs required for ketosis (not coincidentally, they weren't tracking, so it was easy to fudge the numbers and pretend they were sticking with a lower carb count). These "I tried keto, and it didn't work" folks tend to pinball back and forth between their typical diet and keto, too. Which means that they really don't spend much time at all in sustained ketosis or train their body to use fat as its primary fuel source.

I'm all for adding more variety into my diet, eating ice cream once in a while (the full sugar kind) and moving away from strict keto once your goals are achieved. But don't slash your tires then complain that the car doesn't drive correctly. Keto works—but only if you actually DO it.

Most people find that, with actual adherence to the diet, they lose around two pounds a week on keto. Some people have more dramatic initial results (because keto uses a lot of water and electrolytes as you start to use fat for fuel, some of this initial weight loss is water). But between the natural calorie drop-off and the switch from carbs to fat as fuel, consistent weight loss is pretty darn assured for those who follow the diet.

Do I Have to Keto fOrEvER?

I'm gonna point out that most of the people who ask this question are in the initial "adjustment phase" and are feeling the craving for carbs HARD. Your body is playing all kinds of Jedi mind tricks to get you to eat some white bread, and you think about this dismal, breadless future stretching out before you.

I have good news for you: When you adapt to fat and get through that initial un-fun introductory phase, keto is actually very pleasant. Especially as you reach your goals and can incorporate more variety into your diet. Even strict keto, with a little effort, is tasty and fulfilling and even fun.

What I'm saying is, you might surprise yourself by the thought, "Oh wow, I could totally eat like this forever," once you're past the hard stuff at the beginning. It can take between three weeks and around three months to really adjust to keto and transform the way your body uses energy. Stick with it for that long before feeling the "woe is me; do I have to eat like this forever" too hard.

Remember, when you reach your goals there's no reason (except the die-hards on the Internet) you can't slowly add back some of the higher-carb fruits, veggies, and even some whole grains that you've been missing in moderate amounts. Sustainability is more important than perfection. And most people find that they can keep their metabolic flexibility (they can transition easily between fat or carbs) and maintain their health goals even when they increase their carb count. (Smartly!)

Will Keto Raise My Cholesterol?

I was worried about this one. In part because I was still sort of afraid of fat. I mean, it's FAT: the villain in all our foods for our entire lives, if you grew up in the 90s and early 2000s.

"You're gonna clog up your arteries," one of my friends told me knowingly as he popped a bagel bite into his mouth.

So I did all the research I could. Because I wasn't interested in fitting into my pants at all costs. Here's what I learned:

Keto CAN raise your cholesterol. But not in the way you think. Studies show that keto actually LOWERS your LDL (bad) cholesterol while raising your HDL (good) cholesterol. I guess my biggest takeaway here was that I didn't know that much about cholesterol, and neither did my friend who wanted to warn me about clogging up my arteries. Cholesterol (like fat) isn't good or bad. Some cholesterol is actually pretty vital for your health (that's the HDL). And other cholesterol … not so much.

That study I linked isn't the only one out there that has studied the link between fat and cholesterol, and a low-carb diet and cholesterol. At the end of the day, there really isn't any evidence that keto will raise your LDL cholesterol. Most of the reputable studies out there actually show that keto lowers it.

What About My Friend's Dietitian Aunt Who Says Keto is the Devil's Diet?

Fun fact: fiber used to be called the "anti-nutrient." Dietitians saw zero purpose for it and actually went so far as to demonize fiber. They said it would mess up your digestive system and maybe even poison you a little.

In other words, take great care who you listen to. Certainly, there is conflicting and forthcoming information about all KINDS of stuff in the field of nutrition. Remember what the food pyramid looked like? There are still dietitians who insist it was right all along, with that big old base of spaghetti and white bread. Nowadays, almost zero nutritionists agree that the food pyramid should look like this (or even be a pyramid). But for a long time there (while I was in high school) the debates raged hot and heavy over that food pyramid. Why? Because the idea that it was wrong flew in the face of how a lot of people (including nutritionists) saw the world, food, and their own knowledge base.

I trust science. I trust professionals who consult science and are willing to change their stance based on new information. I find that most of the "professionals" who are highly critical of keto actually don't know much about keto when questioned. They have a lot of stereotypes in their head about mayo and bacon—and not much else. The folks I've had a chat with (I got in a long "discussion" with one of my friends who owns a gym and does nutrition coaching) who are willing to listen and learn what keto REALLY is tend to see the diet differently afterward. Keto isn't weird. It isn't a fad. It's getting back to the way our bodies were meant to digest food and process it into energy.

Is Keto Just a Fad?

I hear this question a lot. Keto isn't a fad any more than wearing blue-light glasses is a fad. Yeah, we're newly aware (and by that I mean the general population is newly aware) of the health benefits of low-carb living and the fact that processed foods and sugar are the true public enemy number one when it comes to heart disease (not fat).

It's new. It's popular. (Because people are like "holy shit, I can eat bacon and LOSE WEIGHT and maybe even reverse my pre-hypertension?") But it's not a fad. Our love-affair with "low-fat" and "low-calorie even if it's pure sugar" was a fad. We are now exiting that fad and returning to the way our bodies were meant to digest food. We recognize (thanks, science!) more than ever the importance of gut health. I mean, we had no idea up until a few years ago that 90 PERCENT OF YOUR SEROTONIN and 50 PERCENT OF YOUR DOPAMINE were produced in your gut. And what messes up your gut big-time? Reliance on simple sugars and carbs.

Keto isn't a fad. It's popular. For good reason. And the results speak for themselves.

Won't Saturated Fats Give Me a Heart Attack?

Saturated fats are not the villain you think they are. And they are not the cause of heart attacks. Mounting evidence shows that sugar and processed carbs lead to the inflammation and plaques that cause heart attacks. Numerous studies show that if 25 percent or more of your diet comes from sugar (including stuff like white bread, which is just refined carbs that your body uses as sugar!) you are TWICE as likely to die from a heart attack. Reliance on simple sugars results in inflammation, weight gain, fatty liver disease, and heart disease.

Saturated fats, despite their rep, have not been linked to heart disease and heart attacks.

You're still going to want to avoid trans fats/partially hydrogenated oils on a keto diet (e.g., margarine). Trans fats WILL raise your LDL (bad cholesterol) and can cause other serious health issues.

Like carbohydrates, the best rule of thumb is this: The more processed a fat source (like margarine), the less healthy it is. The less processed (animal fats and nuts), the healthier it generally is.

Animal fats are STILL a cause for concern for other reasons (e.g., the body tends to store pollutants and toxins in fat tissue to protect the internal organs; not to mention issues surrounding cruelty to animals). When you eat animal fats, look for cage-free, grass-fed, cruelty-free, and organic options whenever possible.

Is There Anyone Who SHOULDN'T Do Keto?

Keto is safe for the vast majority of people. HOWEVER, if you are currently struggling with high blood pressure, diabetes, or liver problems (remember, ketones are produced in the liver), you're gonna want medical supervision as your body adjusts to the diet.

If you're pregnant or breastfeeding, a keto diet isn't ideal either. Keto naturally shrinks your calorie intake (while helping you feel fuller), which means that you may not get enough calories for you AND baby while on keto. If you have any questions about your personal situation, be safe and consult a doctor (ideally someone who understands the benefits of a low-carb diet under most circumstances). You'd be surprised how many medical experts are still stuck in the mindset of the old food pyramid, despite the fact that science has unequivocally moved on.

CHAPTER 3
What the Heck Am I Supposed to Eat, Mayo?

Okay, I know that was a lot of questions. But given the villain we've made of fat in our society and the "trendiness" of the keto diet, questions ABOUND.

AKA, before we bother with WHAT to eat, it's really important to understand WHY you're eating it. Otherwise, it's just too scary to dive into those delicious fats.

Are you pumped up? Are you ready to transition your digestive system back to the way nature intended you to consume and create energy? Are you ready to "just say no" to sugar and refined, processed carbs? It's okay if you feel sad about bread. I felt sad about bread for a while. But keep your chin up. We're about to dive into what you CAN eat during a keto diet—without feeling hungry—so buckle up, buttercup. Your mouth is gonna water. I know it.

The hardest part of a keto diet is figuring out what you can eat, so you're full and generally happy with life instead of fantasizing about bread while you try to convince yourself that another avocado will make you feel happy.

There are three requirements for the recipes and food suggestions you'll find in this book: First, they have to taste good. Second, they have to be pretty easy to make. (Nobody has time to be a chef consistently. If you do, congrats to you.) Third, they have to be low carb (duh!).

A-List Foods (Dig in, Baby)

Introducing the new superstars of your diet! This category includes the staples of your diet. You'll notice they're mainly whole, unprocessed foods like nuts, meats, eggs, vegetables, dairy, and some fruit. These are the foods to reach for when you're hungry, when you're planning meals, or when you really need a snack. If you build your diet around these foods and create new meal habits around these foods, your success rate goes WAY up. So, without further ado, here are your go-to foods:

Meats, Fish, and Eggs

The vast majority of meats, fish, and eggs are great choices for keto. Salmon, tuna, lamb, steak, ground beef, chicken, and pork are excellent sources of both fat and protein.

Tip: Don't fall into old habits of choosing "lean meats." Remember, fat is your friend. Not only will higher fat content fill you up faster, but it'll infuse so much more flavor in your meals. (Which means you'll enjoy it more!) Try choosing chicken thighs instead of chicken breast, ribeye instead of sirloin, and salmon instead of tilapia.

Saturated Fats

Saturated fats, as we recently learned, are not the enemy. Don't be afraid to incorporate butter, ghee, lard, coconut oil, and other animal fats into your meals to add flavor (if you haven't eaten Brussels sprouts cooked in bacon grease, you aren't fully alive yet).

Unsaturated Fats

Unsaturated fats (which generally come from plants) are your friend on a keto diet, too. Common unsaturated fats include avocados, olive oil, and sesame oil.

Full-fat Dairy

Skip the "low-fat" options. (You'll find them LOADED with sugar!) Instead, enjoy full-fat yogurt, cream, cottage cheese, cheeses, cream cheese, sour cream. Full-fat milk is also fine in small amounts (just watch that carb count).

For some reason, it was choosing full-fat yogurt that triggered my "But fat is bad" warning bells more than anything else. Maybe because that phrase "low-fat" on the carton had been so deeply tied to my idea of "healthy" for a long time. Thankfully, full-fat dairy tastes way better than the low-fat nonsense.

Nuts and Nut Flours

Nuts are a great source of fat. They're a fantastic keto snack, a superstar in salads, and a good food-on-the-go when needed. Most nuts are pretty high in fat, but keep an eye on pistachios and cashews (these nuts have slightly higher carb counts). Excellent low-carb nuts include almonds, macadamia nuts, pine nuts, pecans, sunflower seeds, pumpkin seeds, flaxseeds, chia seeds, walnuts, and hazelnuts.

Nut FLOURS (made from almond or coconuts) are a fantastic substitute for white flour and can be used to create some of the food staples you might miss (like tortillas and even bread). Cooking with these flours is a little different from white flour, but you'll love the new, delicious recipes (we'll get there later in the book!) and how full you feel from all the fiber.

Non-Starchy Vegetables

Non-starchy veggies are loaded with fiber, micronutrients, and flavor. Keto superstars include broccoli, Swiss chard, cauliflower, kale, peppers, cherry tomatoes, spinach, lettuce, and Brussels sprouts, asparagus, cucumber, zucchini, and summer squash.

Low-Carb Condiments

There's a wide variety of keto-friendly condiments that can spice up your meals and snacks. Gold-star winners include mustard, pesto, mayonnaise, cocoa powder, ranch dressing, Caesar dressing, vinegar, fish sauce, soy sauce, and natural carb-free sweeteners like Stevia and Erythritol. Eat your fill of pickled foods like kimchi, pickles, pickled asparagus, and sauerkraut, too!

The major condiment to watch out for is ketchup. Swap out your old standby with a sugar-free option, because traditional ketchup (and ketchup-based condiments) are packed with carbs.

Low-Carb Beverages

In addition to water (and you're gonna want to drink plenty of water because your body needs it more than ever to create energy with ketones!) you can drink as much as you want of the following beverages: Unsweetened teas (or teas sweetened with stevia), sugar-free soda (there's a raging debate about the healthfulness of sugar-free soda, since it's highly acidic, so proceed with caution and maybe don't drink a gallon a day if you're worried), and coffee.

No more juice or other sugary drinks. Contrary to what you might have been told as a kid, orange juice is NOT a cure-all. Without fiber, you're getting a huge sugar-punch from any kind of juice. Stick to whole fruits instead of juices. If you REALLY need a juice fix, opt for celery juice or lemon-water. (Actually pretty tasty!)

Natural Zero-Calorie Sweeteners

Natural zero-calorie sweeteners like monk fruit powder and stevia can make the diet significantly tastier and more varied. I (and most others) recommend using natural sweeteners instead of erythritol and xylitol, simply because they're easier for your body to recognize as food. There's also been a few studies about those artificial sweeteners causing gut problems (which we're trying to avoid). If you don't tolerate sweeteners well (some people don't), listen to your body and cut them out completely.

B-List Foods (Incorporate These Foods Into Your Meals But Mind Your Portions)

Think of this next group of foods as your supporting cast (if your life were a play and food were the delicious little actors). For any given meal or snack, make the "anytime foods" the star of your plate. But incorporate these secondary foods for variety, micronutrients, and because they taste good!

You'll notice that, like your A-List foods, these B-listers are mainly whole foods—just a little higher in carbohydrates. When you've accomplished your goals (or as your body readjusts to using mostly fat for fuel instead of mostly carbs), you can slowly add more of the higher-carb whole foods to your diet.

Low-Carb Fruit

To make the most of keto, you'll want to choose lower carb fruits. Berries are almost always a safe choice: blackberries, strawberries, cranberries, raspberries, and blueberries. Watermelon, cantaloupe, and honeydew melon are also good choices in moderation. Be careful of apples and tropical fruits like bananas, grapes, and pineapple (these are very high carb; we'll talk about them in the next section).

Semi-Starchy Veggies

There's a number of veggies that can add variety, delicious flavors, and micronutrients to your keto diet. These veggies are a bit starchier and have a higher carb count, but in moderation they're fantastic. Veggies in this category include mushrooms, onions, snap peas, beets, carrots, and sweet potatoes.

High-Fiber, Lower-Carb Whole Grains

You might have heard that grains are totally off-limits while you're doing a keto diet. And if you are trying to LOSE weight (rather than maintain) you're going to want to lay off most grains. However, as you make inroads to your health goals and weight loss goals, you absolutely can add some grains into your diet in moderation for variety (and because they're delicious).

Here are the best options:
- Oats (Half a cup has just 10.5 net carbs)
- Quinoa (half a cup has 17 net carbs)
- Bulgur (half a cup has 12.5 net carbs)
- Wild rice (16 net carbs in a half cup)
- Popcorn (6.5 net carbs in one cup plain, popped)

Seeing a pattern here? All of these grains are whole foods. You're gonna want to steer clear of processed grains that are formed from refined flour and wheat: e.g., crackers, white bread, instant rice, white rice, cereal, pizza crust, and potato chips.

C-List, Supporting Cast Foods (Occasional Treats)

I want to point out right from the start that these foods are all listed here for a reason. And that reason is, they're significantly more processed. They aren't found in nature. And that means your body has a harder time digesting them and extracting energy from them. (Just like white bread!) However, many of them are delicious and can add variety and joy to your diet. These foods aren't bad for that reason alone. But they don't deserve a starring role in every meal.

Keto Bread and Low-Carb Tortillas

Look, I'm a sucker for keto bread. Franz makes this light, airy, fool-you-thinking-it's-white-bread "Keto Bread," and "Keto Buns" that make you feel like you're eating a real sandwich or burger. Same with the tortillas (made by Mission). They're tasty, and they make taco night so much more fun. I buy this stuff often but use it up slowly (they last great in the fridge). Keto buns and bread, and low-carb tortillas are HIGHLY processed despite being delicious. They're franken-foods made of modified wheat starch and oat fiber, along with a long list of other modified ingredients. They're "keto-friendly" because they are essentially ALL fiber, so your net carbs end up being very low.

A quick warning about these foods (especially the bread): They'll make you feel full VERY quickly. Like, one slice. That alone is awesome, just don't down half a loaf or you're gonna be feeling BAD. One guy I read about went to the hospital. Because one slice contains HALF your daily fiber intake.

Again, I use this stuff regularly to add variety and joy to my diet. I can't handle bunless burgers all the time. Sometimes, I just want a regular burger. But I don't eat this stuff for every meal because it's really not a food as much as it is a sort of frankenfood. It's hard on the digestive system, and some people find it spikes their blood sugar (because that whopper fiber content is added, not naturally occurring).

Processed "Keto" Meals, Shakes, and Treats

Be very careful of relying on branded, packaged "keto" treats, shakes, and foods. Unprocessed, whole foods (that don't have a ton of additives and mystery ingredients) are always a better choice for your gut health and overall health.

That said, these foods CAN be super useful in a pinch or on-the-go. After a LOT of experimentation, I recommend the following for taste and texture:

- Atkins frozen meals: The packaging isn't that pretty. But after trying EVERY variety of Atkins frozen meal (and a lot of non-Atkins frozen meals), I'm calling it. Every variety was pretty darn tasty (even the Pork Verde, which sounded super gross to me at first). They're all pretty reasonably low net carb, and on busy days once in a while they're a lifesaver. The shakes and treats are pretty good as well. But watch your portions on the treats. They WILL give you straight-up diarrhea if you eat too many of them.

- Rebel Ice Cream: I'm gonna say it: Some of the treats you'll find out there labeled "keto" are straight-up GROSS and don't taste like anything resembling a "treat," especially ice cream. Rebel has nailed their texture and taste. Pretty much any variety is a solid choice, but particularly the Butter Pecan and the Oreo.

- Breyer's Carb Balance Ice Cream: Again, this stuff tastes so good my kids will eat it (and they are NOTORIOUSLY PICKY). One time I tried to feed them keto pancakes, and they ran from the room.

I know that's a short list, but I'm not going to BS you. Some people LOVE other brands and other prepared keto foods as occasional treats. I'm pretty picky. Explore at will, but don't say I didn't warn you when the mouth-watering image on the package entices you to purchase then leaves you saying, "What the fresh hell is this" as you pop a bite into your mouth.

Alcohol

Alcohol isn't a health food. We all know this (I mean, hopefully we all know this). But sometimes the joy-factor of a drink is worth it. And that's okay. I tend to keep my alcohol use sparing on keto, but when I do want to have a drink, here's what I keep in mind:

First of all, a fair warning: Alcohol will keep your liver busy and will slow ketosis down substantially. But if you ARE going to have a night-cap or a cold one with dinner, opt for dry white or red wine, low-carb beer, or a sugar-free mixed drink with vodka, whiskey, gin, tequila, or rum. (All of them are carb free, but don't get too excited: Remember, they'll slow down ketosis.)

Highly Processed, Preserved Meats

Not to get all high and mighty on you—I love a good hotdog as much as the next girl—but whenever possible choose uncured, unprocessed meats. Enjoy highly processed meats as occasional additions to your diet. That means hot dogs, salami, pepperoni, sausage, and faux meats (these are often loaded with carbs, so watch out).

Remember, the goal here is gut health and getting your body back to basics with energy production and digestion. Processed food always throws a kink in the machine.

Tropical Fruit

This one is hard for me. Tropical fruit is DELICIOUS. But if your goals include losing weight quickly with keto and dealing with health issues, you're going to want to reduce your portions here (especially while you're in go-mode and adjusting to the diet).

Don't get me wrong: These fruits are tasty and packed with good stuff like vitamins and enzymes. But their sugar content will kick you out of ketosis pretty quickly if you consume them often and in larger quantities. So, enjoy these tropical fruits as treats and in smaller quantities. That includes papayas, bananas, mangos, grapes, and pineapple. Anything that grows in warm, tropical climates.

Vegetable Oils

You're going to want to limit the hydrogenated and partially hydrogenated oils, corn oil, canola oil, vegetable oil, and margarine for the same reason you cut down on processed meats. They're not great for your body, they're hard to digest, and they aren't good fuel for your health goals.

Black-Listed Foods (You'll Never Work in This Town AGAIN!)

You should cut these foods out of your life and diet as much as possible. There's really no redeeming nutritional value here, and they can actually hurt your digestive system and gum up the works. Lame.

But real talk? Some of these foods are delicious. And we can't ignore the joy factor that comes from eating them. As you reach your goals and adjust to keto, you're going to find your cravings disappear for the most part. You aren't going to feel like you'd kill a man for a Dairy Queen Blizzard every night anymore. But … sometimes ice cream will still sound good. And that's okay. Sometimes a keto treat doesn't cut it. I just want you to rest assured right here that we WILL cover "cheating" later in the book. I'm pro-cheat, as part of a sustainable approach to diet. I've found it helps me stay more consistent and commit to a way of life rather than a white-knuckle approach. But we'll get to that later. For now, while you adapt, nix all of the following foods:

Sugar

Ah, sugar. This is a big one. Sugar is addictive, easy energy (even if it completely wreaks havoc on your digestive system at the same time), and your body can easily become addicted to it. Your body will protest when you cut out sugar. It will give you cravings like a drug user. Which makes sense, because sugar hijacks your brain in a similar way to some drugs and encourages dependence despite its harm.

Basically, giving up sugar is rough. But, like giving up drugs, it gets easier. Expect withdrawals. Like, intense withdrawals. But hang in there knowing they WILL get better after a few days and disappear after a few weeks.

You'll want to avoid all forms of sugar, including refined cane sugar, agave, honey, artificial sweeteners (like Equal and Splenda), ice cream, pastries, and soda. Keep in mind that many products hide high levels of sugar. (Like ketchup!) Check those labels when in doubt.

Juice

A lot of us grew up thinking that juice was fruit in a bottle. Especially if it was "100 percent juice." Unfortunately, juice (even natural juice) is highly processed and devoid of any fiber. (Which mitigates all that sugar!) Juice is PACKED with sugar. Eat fruit, not juice. It's sugar. Fight me.

White or Wheat Flour

White or wheat flour is a highly refined source of carbs that just isn't great for you or your digestive system. I know it's delicious. But it's not a good source of energy or good for your gut. And it'll kick you right out of ketosis. Stay away from pasta, pizza crust, bread, etc. Anything made from white flour (or wheat flour).

That's the rundown on foods. When in doubt, look at carb count and fiber to determine your net carbs. Fill your plate with A-list foods, supplement with B-list and then C-list foods for variety and deliciousness, and treat yourself with the black-balled foods on occasion if they bring you joy. Do that, and you're well on your way to success and reaching your goals with keto!

CHAPTER 4

Tracking and Getting Results: Exactly How Many Carbs Can I Eat and Still Lose Weight?

Let's be honest: Tracking food is obnoxious. It can feel like one more thing that makes you say, "Screw it, I'm eating chips," at the end of a hard day.

Track anyway.

Not forever. But for the first little while as you are adapting to keto, adapting to using fat for energy, and breaking your addiction to sugar and refined carbohydrates. Why? A few reasons:

1. It's really, really easy to think to yourself, "I bet there are not that many carbs in this …" (as you down your entire day's worth of carbs). Your brain will try to trick you into eating carbohydrates. Especially the refined, sugary, white-floury ones it's addicted to. Suddenly, you'll be thinking, "Just one Cheez-It can't have that many carbs. I'll just eat one … or two … I mean, that's not even a serving." Don't do it. Don't let your brain trick you into dragging out your reliance on processed carbs.

2. Tracking carbs is a lot different from tracking calories. There is NO need to go hungry while tracking carbs. Even if you've hit your daily allotment for carbohydrates, you can ALWAYS eat a zero-carb snack. (Like an egg!) Giving your body the option to eat when it's hungry—while restricting carbs—is a fascinating exercise. You might at first think, "Man, I'm starving." But nothing but carbs sound good to you. That's your brain trying to be sneaky. You'll find that when you are ACTUALLY hungry, fats and protein and fiber sound good: you know, real fuel. Not just a sugar rush.

45

3. Tracking helps you stay accountable to your goals and KNOW whether you are on track to succeed. If you guess, you won't really know. And you certainly won't be able to say "Yeah, I tried keto, but it didn't work for me." If you're going to do keto, do keto. There is no try. (Say that in Yoda's voice, please.)
4. Creating new habits with food is challenging. And you might be surprised by which foods contain a whopper-load of carbs. Use tracking as an opportunity to get familiar with which foods are A-list, B-list, and C-list in your diet.

You don't need to track your food forever. But I HIGHLY recommend it during the first three weeks of your introduction to a keto diet, while you adjust. After that, you'll be very familiar with your go-to foods, their carb count, and how it feels to adapt to using fat for energy.

My favorite tool for counting carbs is Carb Manager. It's a free app, and it counts carbs first and calories second. Aka, you'll know your calorie count. But it won't be the main focus of the app. Carb Manager has a pretty exhaustive database of foods, and you can easily copy and create meals to save time on tracking.

Okay, So How Many Carbs Can I Eat?

We covered this question a bit in the introduction, but the short answer is that most people need to stay under 30 grams of net carbs for maximum results.

That said, every person is different. You know that. Some people can go up to 50 grams of carbs and still lose weight or reach their health goals rapidly. Your magic number will vary, and if you want to experiment I recommend waiting until AFTER the three-week introduction to keto before you go off-grid.

With just 30 grams of net carbs per day, your calorie intake is going to naturally drop pretty low (even while you feel full). You won't get many insulin spikes (because carbohydrates trigger those) that signal your body to store sugar as fat. And between the naturally low-calorie threshold and the low carb count, your body is going to start dipping into its own fat stores as it shifts to relying on consumed and stored fat for energy.

If you have a lot of weight to lose (e.g., a lot of stored fuel for your body to access), you can comfortably stay in this zone for a while until you reach your weight goals. How long you stay in this ultra-low-carb zone depends on how much stored fat you've got to supplement your consumed fat.

As you reach your goals, you'll likely want to increase your carb count (and calorie count through whole-food carbs to between 50 and 100 grams a day). Why? Because if your body is in low-calorie, no-fat-stores mode, you run the risk of lowering your basal metabolic rate. Essentially, your body recognizes that you don't have enough consumed fat or stored fat and tries to conserve energy as much as possible to avoid starving (by doing things like lowering your body temperature, slowing down digestion, etc.). And we don't want that. We want a body that can be flexible in how it consumes energy, has a healthy gut, and plenty of fuel for all its functions.

Optimizing Keto for Weight Loss

If you're primarily in the market to fit back in your pants (I get it, been there), I'm going to share a few tried-and-true strategies to make sure you get what you need from the keto diet:

First of all, let's get your mindset right: You CAN do this. You are not doomed to buy bigger pants year after year. Numerous studies show that a low-carb, high-fat diet is highly effective when it comes to weight loss.

And again, keto might sound strange at first, but it's actually the easiest diet to lose weight, for a lot of reasons. For one thing, you can EAT when you are HUNGRY. (You just can't eat endless carbs.) So, there's no stress in starving yourself. For another thing, you're going to find that your blood sugar stabilizes. There's no white-knuckled, "hangry" crashes or rollercoaster energy levels. With a sustainable, accessible source of energy (fat) cravings for sugar disappear, replaced by a sense of satiety that allows you to eat only when hungry.

Here are my best tips for using keto to lose weight:

Don't Pay too Much Attention to Calories

ESPECIALLY when starting out, avoid counting calories and focus on your body's hunger signals. Eat when you're hungry, stop as soon as you're full, and stick to the diet (that last part is IMPORTANT). Before you get hung up on restricting calories, make sure you are actually counting your carbs. You don't need to go hungry. You just need to stick to your carb counts.

Eat Enough Protein

Make sure your protein intake isn't falling short of 15 percent or in excess of 30 percent. Protein helps you feel full, and it helps you preserve and build muscle mass (critical for weight loss and general health). Too little protein, and you're going to feel hungry. Too much protein, and your body is gonna convert that excess into storage.

Find Your Magic Carb Number

If you are SURE you are being diligent in counting your carbs, and you aren't losing weight, you might need to lower your carb count a bit to really maximize ketosis. Everyone's a little different when it comes to carb tolerance. While you'll definitely want to keep carb intake below 50 grams of net carbs per day, many people find that reducing carbohydrate intake to 20 grams of net carbs per day, especially during the initial months of a keto diet, can dramatically improve weight loss.

Watch that Carb Creep!

Remember, especially during the first month, your brain is trying to sneak carbs. Don't nibble without counting, don't eat "sugar-free" foods without counting, don't "cheat" without counting and then tell yourself keto "didn't work for you." It will work, but only if you're honest with yourself! Even small amounts of carbohydrates can make a big difference over time when you add them up over the course of a day.

Eat MCTs (Medium-Chain Triglycerides)

Adding more medium-chain triglycerides—most commonly coconut oil —to your diet can help improve weight loss during a ketogenic diet. MCTs are easy to digest, unlikely to be stored as additional fat, and encourage ketone production in the liver (ketones help you convert stored fat into energy).

Eat Real Foods

Take a close look at the type of calories you're consuming. Are you eating real, unprocessed foods that align with the macronutrient percentages of a keto diet? If not, readjust and realign. Real foods that your body recognizes are going to fuel positive results no matter what your goals.

Stay Realistic

It's important to stay positive and remember that weight loss isn't a straightforward process. Try not to gauge your success in terms of a number on a scale, but rather in how your clothes fit and how your body composition changes.

Balance Your Carb Count in Meals and Snacks

Your goal should be to balance your macros each time you eat. E.g., you don't want to eat all fat for breakfast and lunch, then your entire day's worth of carbs at dinner. That might sound satisfying, but it'll give you a huge insulin spike at dinner and throw your body into a bit of a tailspin (and intensify your old cravings). Try to balance your carbs, fat, and protein at EVERY meal. And keep snacks protein- or fat-based (rather than carb-based).

Remember the Stress and Sleep Factors

Losing the max amount of weight with the keto diet is tied to several other important factors, including your stress level. Stress is directly correlated to an uptick in cortisol, which facilitates fat storage. In other words, try to relax and embrace the process!

How much sleep you're getting each night is important too. Sleep quality is directly tied to hormone production, organ health, and digestive health. Don't slash your tires by getting poor sleep while you're trying to accomplish this task.

How Much Weight Can I Expect to Lose?

I can't give you a golden number. But can I tell you that, on average, between the calorie deficit and a much healthier relationship with your digestive system, you are likely to lose between one and five pounds per week. That depends A LOT on how much weight you have to lose (the more weight you have to lose, the quicker it tends to come off) and how well you follow your carb counts.

Here are a few things to keep in mind as you work toward weight loss goals:

Expect Fluctuation

You should expect some fluctuations as your body adjusts. Expect to retain water periodically (your fat cells will fill up with water as your body uses that fat as fuel, as your body tries to gauge whether you still need a placeholder to store additional fat). There's no need to worry though. As you rein in your carb intake, your body will release stored glycogen and temporary water weight.

Be Patient

If your body has been accustomed to relying on carbohydrates and sugars for a long time, expect an adjustment period and some fluctuation in weight. Be kind to yourself and patient with your body as you work toward your goals, and remember that your body may just need some time to adjust to the keto diet before you see results.

Consider Your Target Weight

As you reach your target weight, your pace of weight loss is going to slow down. That's normal, and that means you're running out of excess storage. That's fantastic! Don't push it beyond your healthy weight: Your body won't like it and may even try to slow your metabolism to protect what's left of your storage. Pay attention to your body's signals, your body's composition of fat and muscle, and take your health into key consideration as you decide whether or not you want to push beyond a particular weight plateau.

CHAPTER 5
Getting Through the First Three Weeks, AKA "Keto Hell"

I've already mentioned it a couple of times, but it's worth repeating (in fact, it's worth a whole chapter): The first three weeks are pretty hard.

You need to think of that first stretch as a detox. Your body, if it's been pretty reliant on sugar and highly processed carbs, is not going to be in a good place when you take away that supply.

The biggest thing I want you to remember is this: Feeling bad during this detox period is not an indication of any of the following:

- That you will feel like this forever
- That keto was a bad idea
- That something is wrong
- That you are hurting your health

Again, if you had been leading a totally sedentary life for the past year and suddenly tried to run a mile? It would feel awful. That doesn't mean running is bad for you. Or if you decided to stop smoking cigarettes or taking cocaine. Would you feel awful? Yup. Would it last forever? Nope. Would you be healthier and happier after you got through the hard part? Yep.

A LOT of people who try keto quit during the first few days. Which is like starting to roll a big rock up a hill and then letting it roll back down right before you reach the top. KEEP PUSHING, BABY! Because when you get to the top, the going is a lot easier. This chapter is meant to be read while you are in the depths of those first three days. I just need you to know right now that no matter how much you want a big ice cream sundae, you're going to get through this. And you won't want one in the same way a few days from now.

Let's talk about what you can do to get through those first three weeks with as minimal discomfort and distress as possible. There's no way around it: It's gonna feel kinda bad. But life on the other side is better. Here's how you make it through:

Make a Meal Plan, Prep and Shop BEFORE You Dive In

Don't wait until you feel weak and sort of blah and are battling intense carb cravings to plan out your meals, snack options, drink options, and treat options. You need ALL of these things ready to go, because if you don't, that's where your sneaky little brain will target its "Come on, this is too hard, let's just go get some fries" campaign.

Make a shopping list, make a meal plan (even if you're not a planner), knowing that it will save you in your weak moments. You'll find a two-week meal plan and shopping list for this very purpose in this book.

Being hungry during those first few days (like, actually hungry, not just hungry for carbs) is a danger zone you want to avoid at all costs. Fill your fridge, your cupboards, and your pantry with keto-friendly foods (see the previous chapter) that sound good to you and will give you enough variety to last you a week without going back to the store.

Again, you need MEALS, SNACKS, TREATS, and DRINKS. Spend twenty minutes thinking it through. Write down your plan using a basic Google doc, spreadsheet, or just a piece of paper. Then put it somewhere you can access it, so that when you get hungry or think about your next meal, you don't panic. You won't have to do this forever. But you WILL need to do it while your body adjusts and tries to sabotage you into thinking that keto is too hard.

In addition to meal planning, I'm gonna need you to donate or chuck your carby favorites. Don't set yourself up for temptation by keeping chips, cookies, white bread, etc. lying around or in the fridge. If you absolutely MUST keep stuff like this around (e.g., you have picky kids who aren't interested in joining your keto journey), try allocating it to a particular shelf in the pantry or fridge, so you can avoid eye contact.

Plan for Weak Moments

It's going to happen. You're going to feel "meh." You're going to crave carbs something fierce during that adjustment period.

Plan for it. Start the diet with a buddy who will help keep you on track when you're feeling blah. That could be a spouse, a friend from a keto support group on social media, or a sibling. Anyone. As long as they're someone you can turn to (who won't tell you to just give in and eat the fries). A little nudge of support and accountability can be a big help.

I'd also recommend that you create a mini self-care emergency pack for yourself that you can draw from when you're feeling bummed out and the going is hard during that adjustment period. Here are some ideas of what you might include:

- Some fun new keto-friendly snacks
- A new book you've been excited to read
- Bath bombs
- An encouraging note from your spouse or a friend (Ask them to write this before you start keto, and don't read it until you need it!)
- An adult coloring book or another soothing craft you enjoy

Make a pact with yourself that you will NOT quit while you are hungry. Sign a contract if you need to and display it in a visible location. Your contract might say something like, "I will not make a decision about whether to continue with my goals while I am hungry. I will eat a keto-friendly delicious meal before I make any decisions."

Just remember that your risk of quitting goes up exponentially when you are hungry, especially during that adjustment period. Make sure you are stocked up on keto-friendly foods, have a list of go-to snacks and easy meals (we'll talk about all of that!), and keep yourself well-fed. Our goal is not to starve. Our goal is to eat in a new way. And staying well-fed will help you stay the course and avoid weak moments.

Make It as Easy on Yourself as Possible

There will be time for gourmet keto meals. And if that's how you roll or you just LOVE to cook intricate stuff, go for it. But for most people, keeping meals and snacks and routines as simple as possible while you adjust to eating in a new way will drastically increase your odds of success. It can be really intimidating to make a time-consuming meal from scratch if you're already feeling weak and hungry and fresh out of motivation. An easy meal can save your goals and your sanity while you adjust.

Simplify wherever you can during this adjustment phase—not just with food. It's probably not the best time to start a high-intensity workout class or learn to play the guitar. Be realistic about the fact that you might not feel your best while your body adapts, and be protective of your time and your obligations. You're doing hard work and making big changes. Keep things as simple as possible for the best chance of success.

And that brings us to my next tip . . .

Don't Start During a High-Stress Time of Life or the Holidays

There's no "good time" to start a new diet or routine. There's always going to be little stresses or minor holidays. But trying to start keto the day after your husband leaves you, or your dog dies, or on Thanksgiving or Christmas will add extra hurdles. And you don't need extra hurdles. Because we want to set ourselves up for the BEST chance of success possible.

So, be honest with yourself in gauging your overall stress level in life. And if you're in a reasonably good place, tally ho! If you're not, it's okay to wait just a little bit.

That said . . .

Accept that There's Never a Good Time to Start

There is always going to be SOMETHING you could use as a reason to wait "just a little longer" to start keto. I get it. It's a little intimidating. It's new. And will it be horrible? (No, but it will be a little challenging, and you are UP to the challenge.)

There's never going to be a perfect time to change your life. Don't let yourself start on Christmas Day. But don't let yourself wait "just one more week" before you dive in and make positive changes to your health and your life in general. Make a plan, choose a start date within the week (so you have time to grocery shop and meal plan) and then stick to it. Don't cancel because of family dinners, social outings, minor holidays, or minor stress. Those things will always be there.

Prioritize your health. Get started. You'll be glad you did.

Plan for Eating Out and Social Situations

We'll really dive into good restaurant go-to's on keto, as well as fast food options later on. Suffice it to say that if you're just getting started, you should plan for restaurants and social gatherings with food BEFOREHAND.

Look at the menu and decide what you'll eat BEFORE someone is passing you the "free" bread at the table. Decide how you'll respond BEFORE when someone asks why you're eating a bunless burger. ("Because I'm fancy and this is a deconstructed, minimalist burger.")

You can wing it later on, when you know your go-to options and are more comfortable passing on the bread (and aren't in deep withdrawals). During your first three weeks, make a plan rather than relying on your wits in the moment (they are no match for that bread when you're adjusting).

Make It Enjoyable

I know that diet culture is tied to suffering in our culture. It makes sense. You suffer in most diets. You can't eat what you want, you can't eat enough to feel full, and you feel bad the whole time.

Despite the fact that these first three weeks are hard (carb withdrawals are HARD, there's no way around it), most people are pleasantly surprised by how different the keto diet feels from other diets. For one thing, you can eat when you're hungry (you just can't eat carbs). For another, a lot of truly delicious foods (like bacon and cheese) are now on the table.

My advice to you is to make as much delicious, enjoyable food as you can during those first three weeks in particular. Eat when you're hungry. Make easy meals that you are looking forward to. Don't punish yourself or behave like this is just another diet full of hunger pangs and deprivation. Identify the foods you really love, and then eat them! Eat the bacon. Eat the cheese. Try some yummy keto treats as you crave them. Find what you love in your new repertoire of foods, and dig in!

You're never going to stick with this diet if you don't enjoy what you're eating. So make it a point to enjoy your meals and your snacks.

Find Non-Food-Based Rewards and Routines

I learned pretty quickly with keto how often I was using sugar and carbs as a quick dopamine hit/sugar rush when I was feeling bored, tired, lonely, or bummed out. When I didn't have that option, I realized that I wasn't even hungry (because I was not remotely interested in a carb-free or low-carb snack).

I had to learn new go-to pick-me-ups that didn't revolve around food. And you will too, for your best chance of success. Some of those options might include 5-minute meditation, reading a chapter of a new book, going for a walk, watching cat videos on TikTok, stretching, sitting on the porch with your spouse and talking while you sip on some keto lemonade (I'll give you the recipe for that later in the book!), or working on a craft or art project for a few minutes. Figure out what small things can give you a little boost or relax you during the day—aside from eating a handful of potato chips or candy.

Having those go-to rewards and routines for yourself in place will help you more easily skirt around carb cravings. It'll also give you a healthier relationship with food by encouraging you to eat when you're truly hungry.

CHAPTER 6
How to Tell Whether
You're in Ketosis

Big question that you may not have considered if you're new to keto: How does one KNOW they are in ketosis?

The first thing to know is that ketosis (when your body actually transitions to using fat for fuel) is not a light switch. It's more of a water faucet. And the fact is, that faucet turns on and off for all of us every day. Otherwise, you'd die when you slept for eight hours without consuming any new energy. Most of us enter MILD ketosis, where that faucet turns on to a trickle and we start dipping into our fat stores just a teensy bit.

Keto turns up the faucet more fully, allowing us to access fat stores more readily and easily.

But again, how will you know you're really turning the faucet on? There's four main ways.

Four Ways to Tell You're in Ketosis

Here's the big four:

Pee Sticks

This is my personal favorite because it's kind of fun.

Keto test strips can be purchased in bulk, very cheaply. They will tell you how much the faucet is turned on by the color of the strip after you pee on it for a few seconds. A few things to be aware of:

> 1. You're likely to get stronger readings early on in your adjustment period. Your body is still gauging its ketone volume and will overproduce when it realizes you're serious about cutting carbs. Expect deeper purple readings at first when you

are consistent with your macros. Don't worry if the readings turn lighter purple over time. As long as you're meeting your macros and getting a positive pee test, you're good to go.

2. These pee strips expire, and they are sensitive to air. So seal up the bottle tight in the cabinet, and toss them when they expire (you'll have a good couple of years, no worries).

Blood Tests

I'll be honest, I've never done this one. I've heard it's pretty darn accurate, and the method is similar to testing blood sugar if you have diabetes. The prick is tiny. And the results are accurate. But I've never been willing to gain that accuracy by drawing blood. If you are, a test meter will last you a long time and provide good results. You'll want to stay in the ketone range of .5-3.0 mmol/L. The higher your reading, the higher that faucet is turned up.

Keto Breath and Pee

In the early stages of your adjustment to a keto lifestyle, you'll notice that your breath has a "fruitier" aroma. Some people think it smells sort of like nail polish. Either way, it's weird and gross but WILL indicate you're in ketosis. Also, it WILL go away as your body adjusts.

Some people also notice stronger-smelling urine as they expel more electrolytes. You may also find that you are thirstier and craving salt more often (more evidence that you're using up more electrolytes than usual.)

Breathalyzer

Breathalyzers: Not just for drunk people! They're also a method for measuring ketones. I'd recommend AGAINST using this method (even though it's kind of cool). Breath strips aren't as accurate as pee strips, and you have to purchase an expensive breath analyzer. Still, some people love the convenience, and it WILL give you a decent baseline. So if you really want one, go for it!

Struggling to Get Into Ketosis? Don't Panic

If you're sticking to the diet (for real) and seeing only faint readings, don't panic. Stay the course. Readings aren't everything. And the little pee sticks can only tell you so much. That said, there is a good way to give your body a boost in producing ketones: BHB (Beta-Hydroxybutyrate) supplements (not to be confused with GHB . . . which is a party drug).

BHB Supplements or Exogenous Ketones

Your body actually produces BHB naturally. Like we learned earlier, these ketones allow your body to break down fat and turn it into energy.

You can give your ketone levels a boost by taking exogenous ketone supplements. "Exogenous" simply means "outside." So, instead of relying on the ketones you produce, you give your liver a break and add some ketones into the mix to help you use fat as energy more easily.

There are a few ketone supplements on the market, and I don't really care to recommend any of them in particular because in my opinion they're all pretty darn similar in effectiveness. However, some taste better than others and we'll get to that in a sec.

BHB supplements can help you essentially turn up the faucet of ketosis, allowing you to burn fat more rapidly and ease symptoms of the "keto flu" (the withdrawal period as you adjust to removing the bulk of carbs from your diet). Many keto newbies choose to supplement with BHB to make the adjustment period easier.

BHB can also help you return to ketosis more quickly after you "cheat" or eat a higher-carb meal. It's just not realistic to stay in ketosis all the time. But BHB can help you return to a state of ketosis more smoothly without another adjustment period if you hop off the rails for a bit.

Options for Ketone Supplements: Pills, Drinks, and Powders

You can find BHB supplements in three different forms: pills, powders, and drinks. Ketones don't naturally taste AWESOME, so pills are a popular choice for good reason. They're also quite discreet, so if you don't want to alert your coworkers that you are K-E-T-O, this is a good option. Don't ignore the suggested dosage on the pills. They'll give you diarrhea.

Powders and pre-mixed drinks are typically more expensive than pills, but many of them make a handy meal substitute and taste pretty decent. Check out reviews before you buy, and purchase in sample sizes when possible to find flavors that you like.

CHAPTER 7
Easy Beverages
That Legitimately Taste Good

With the mechanics, questions, and pitfalls out of the way, it's time to dive into the fun stuff: Recipes. I solemnly swear to include only recipes I have tried (and enjoyed) PERSONALLY. Every recipe in this book is easy, tastes good, and has been personally vetted. One of my top frustrations when starting keto was the huge range of recipe quality out there. Some stuff looked AMAZING in photos and tasted like garbage. And some stuff just took so long to make that it wasn't worth the stress.

I'm starting with beverages, because that's my first go-to in the morning (you know I'm talking about coffee). But staying hydrated is VERY important on a keto diet. You're using a ton of electrolytes, and you are adjusting to a new way of eating. Your body needs to be hydrated and primed to roll with the carb withdrawals.

Creamy Keto Americano

This Americano is rich, creamy, and absolutely delicious. Using heavy cream not only gives you a full-bodied flavor (unlike skim milk), but you score just one gram of net carbs and only 100 calories. Pour over ice for a cold, refreshing option!

   2 shots espresso
   6 oz. hot water
   2 Tb. heavy whipping cream
   Stevia or sugar-free syrup to taste (I prefer the Davinci brand sugar-free Vanilla, White Chocolate, and Toasted Marshmallow flavors, but there are LOADS to choose from. Your typical grocery store will have a

limited selection, but look for a local restaurant supply store for better selection, or order from Amazon.)

Mix all ingredients in a mug until stevia is dissolved and enjoy.

Net carbs: 1

Keto Coconut Latte

Generally, you'll want to skip milk with your coffee. But coconut milk is a notable exception and makes this latte taste amazing! Make sure you opt for the "unsweetened" coconut milk. And 40 calories for a latte? That's magic, my friend.

2 shots espresso
8 oz. unsweetened Silk coconut milk
Stevia or sugar-free syrup to taste.

Mix all ingredients in a mug until stevia is dissolved and enjoy.

Net carbs: 1

Keto Mocha Latte

Generally, you'll want to skip milk with your coffee. But coconut milk is a notable exception and makes this latte taste amazing! Make sure you opt for the "unsweetened" coconut milk. And 40 calories for a latte? Yes, please!

2 shots espresso
1 Tb. unsweetened baking cocoa
8 oz. unsweetened Silk coconut milk
Stevia or sugar-free syrup to taste.

Mix the baking cocoa with the espresso while it's still warm. Then add the coconut milk and stevia in a mug. Voila! Chocolatey!

Net carbs: 2

Keto Tea

Really any herbal tea, black tea, or green tea is going to be zero-carb and keto-friendly. (Just make sure that if you purchase pre-made tea, it's not the sweetened kind.)

Turn your favorite flavor tea into something special by adding a tablespoon of heavy cream and some stevia for just 1 gram of net carbs and 50 calories. I love the Nutty Almond Relaxer herbal tea by Tiesta; it tastes like apple pie in a cup and is bright pink! For black tea, anything by Twinings and Celestial seasonings is superb!

Chocolate Banana Keto Breakfast Smoothie

This smoothie is a little carbier, so make sure you ONLY use ¼ banana (seriously, stick to just 1/4th). Bananas pack a carb punch, but they're a great source of potassium, and I'm personally unwilling to give up the flavor and texture they add to my smoothies in favor of sad cauliflower.) That said, you CAN substitute ¼ cup cauliflower into this recipe to bring the net carb count to 3. Some people swear they can't taste the cauliflower, and it does give you that banana-y texture. I'm just picky.

¼ banana (or ¼ C. cauliflower to save 6 net carbs)
1 Tb. unsweetened baking cocoa
1 serving low-carb chocolate protein powder (I like the Isopure Dutch Chocolate, but there are lots of good ones.)
1 C. coconut milk
1 tsp. vanilla extract
1 C. of ice (or more, if you want it thicker)
Stevia to taste

Blend all ingredients until smooth.

Net carbs: 9

Keto Lemonade

This stuff is EXCELLENT for sipping throughout the day to keep electrolyte levels high and maintain good hydration. It's especially helpful during your adjustment period to ward off headaches and muscle aches and other symptoms of the temporary "keto flu."

8 oz. ice water
¼ tsp. Salt
1 fresh squeezed lemon (or 2 TB. lemon juice)
Stevia drops to taste

Serve over ice.

Net carbs: 0

Keto Cherry or Strawberry Limeade

I drink this all day. It's delicious, and it's zero calorie and zero carb:

1 Tb. lime juice
1 squirt strawberry or cherry Mio (Or the generic brand, it doesn't matter. If you don't know what this is, it's the little squirt bottle concentrates. You'll find them on the aisle with the Kool-Aid and soda usually.)

Serve over ice.

Net carbs: 0

Keto Italian Soda

This is a great treat that can hit the right notes if you're craving a milkshake:

1 Tb. heavy cream
8 oz. sparkling water
Sugar-free syrup to taste (I like vanilla, coconut, and cherry the best. But choose what you like!)

Serve over ice.

Net carbs: 1

Keto Root Beer Float

Root beer floats are best when the ice cream gets all melty anyway! If you don't mind a few carbs, you can also make a "real" float with Breyer's Carb Smart Ice Cream. (Or another low-carb brand. This one beats them all in terms of texture in my opinion though.)

> 8 oz. diet root beer over ice
> 1 Tb. heavy cream
>
> Serve over ice
>
> Net carbs: 1

Keto Strawberry Watermelon Smoothie

This drink is so refreshing. It's a little carbier but makes a fantastic treat.

> ½ C. watermelon
> ½ C. frozen strawberries
> 1 Tb. lime juice
> 1 squirt Strawberry Watermelon Mio (or another zero-calorie liquid drink concentrate)

Blend until smooth. Add a little water if too thick or a little stevia if not sweet enough for you. This recipe is a bit carbier, so you may want to avoid it during your adjustment phase. But given that most smoothies pack around 60-100 grams of carbs, this one is pretty darn light!

> Net carbs: 9.5

Keto Sex on the Beach

Again, alcohol isn't GOOD for ketosis. It's not good for your liver either. But the joy factor of a drink with friends or after a long day is sometimes worth it. And these drinks pack a very low-carb punch. So if you're going to drink, drink one of them. (Or a low-carb light beer or dry white wine. But you don't need a recipe for that.)

1 shot vodka
½ C. light orange juice
1 Tb. sugar-free strawberry syrup
4 oz. sparkling water

Mix and serve over ice.

Net carbs: 6

Keto Whiskey Diet

This recipe is almost so simple it isn't worth including. But whiskey is zero-carb and makes a nice little drink mixed with Diet Coke or Diet Dr. Pepper.

Keto Margarita

It's 5:00 somewhere. And this marg is a worthy celebration.

1 shot tequila
1 Tb lime
½ C. frozen strawberries
6 oz. sparkling water or fruity diet soda
Stevia to taste

Blend ingredients until smooth, then enjoy with a salt rim (and maybe a fancy little umbrella!)

Net carbs: 2.5

Keto Sparkling Pina Colada

You can't bet this for a low-carb colada. Just mix all ingredients and serve over ice!

1 can Smirnoff Spiked Pina Colada seltzer
1 Tb. sugar-free pineapple syrup
1 Tb. heavy cream

CHAPTER 8
Easy Breakfasts
That Legitimately Taste Good

Breakfast is, in my opinion, the easiest keto meal. You've got SO many great low-carb options at your fingertips. So let's explore some of the yummiest, easiest options!

Keto Chocolate Chip Pancakes/Waffles

So, first things first: You can absolutely find a ton of recipes that include coconut flour or almond flour to make almost any kind of baked good on keto. I don't love the taste of either. If you do, you'll find a plethora of recipes online! I prefer CarbQuik (high fiber carbalose flour). The taste and texture (for me) is far more similar to normal pancakes. You can purchase a bulk container of it on Amazon, and it'll last you a good long time.

1 C. CarbQuik
½ C. water
¼ C. heavy cream
½ stick melted butter
1 egg, beaten
¼ C. dark chocolate chips
Vegetable oil or coconut oil spray

Combine all ingredients except chocolate chips, and mix batter just enough to combine. Spray a griddle or frying pan well, and pour approximately ¼ cup of batter per pancake. Sprinkle chocolate chips on top, and flip when bubbles appear and pop on top of the pancakes. These are delicious plain, or with butter and sugar-free maple syrup. You can make a batch ahead, save it in the fridge, and eat them all week! Note: You can also make these in a waffle iron.

Yields: 10 pancakes
Net carbs per pancake: 2

Keto Biscuits and Gravy

These babies are a LITTLE carbier, but they are worth it. They're easy to make and easy to save for future breakfasts in the fridge.

2 C. CarbQuik
⅔ C. water
3/4 pound Jimmy Dean pork sausage (or your favorite breakfast sausage, just keep an eye on the carb count)
1.5 C. half and half
1 tsp. garlic powder
Salt and pepper to taste
Cooking spray

Reserve 1/8th cup CarbQuik. Combine remaining CarbQuik and water until dough forms. Dough should be smooth but sticky and hold together. Spray a baking sheet and drop spoonfuls of dough onto the baking sheet. Bake at 350 for 10-12 minutes. While biscuits are baking, cook sausage fully. Once browned and crumbled, sprinkle with reserved CarbQuik, then stir in half and half, garlic powder, and salt and pepper. Cook until mixture thickens slightly (about 5 minutes), stirring constantly. Serve warm sausage gravy over biscuits.

Servings: 8
Net carbs per serving: 7

Keto Salsa Verde Breakfast Burrito

My favorite keto tortillas are the Mission Carb Balance Tortillas. They taste just like the real thing, at just four net carbs. They make a fantastic, easy breakfast in this burrito!

1 Mission Carb Balance Tortilla

2 Tb. cheddar cheese
1 oz. sausage, browned then scrambled with 2 eggs
2 Tb. green salsa
1 Tb. sour cream

Low broil the tortilla with cheese sprinkled on top until cheese is melted. Top with sausage and egg scramble, salsa, and sour cream. Add avocado or guac if you wish!

Servings: 1

Net carbs: 6

Keto Veggie Omelette

4 eggs
1 Tb. heavy cream
4 Tb. cheddar
2 Tb. chopped green onions
1 tsp. butter
½ C. chopped fresh mushrooms
1 medium tomato, diced
1 avocado, diced

Sauté mushrooms and green onions with butter at medium heat until mushrooms are golden and tender. Turn down heat to low. Whisk eggs and cream until frothy and pour over mushroom mixture. Cook until egg begins to solidify, then sprinkle cheddar cheese on top. When cheese has melted, fold omelet in half and cook each side until desired doneness. Serve with fresh tomatoes and avocado.

Servings: 4

Net carbs per serving: 2.5

Keto Bacon Spinach Frittata

5 slices bacon
1 Tb. butter

7 C. fresh spinach
8 eggs
1.5 C. shredded cheddar
1 C. heavy cream
1 tsp. garlic powder
1/4 tsp. salt
⅛ tsp. pepper

Grease a 9 x 9 baking dish and preheat oven to 350. Cook bacon until crispy, then set aside and crumble. Add fresh spinach to the pan with the bacon grease, add the butter, and cook until spinach is wilted. Set spinach aside with bacon. Whisk eggs and cream together until fluffy, then pour into the greased pan. Sprinkle the bacon and spinach over the eggs, then top with the cheddar cheese. Cook for 25 minutes, or until eggs have set. Super easy to double and reheat for multiple meals!

Servings: 4

Net carbs per serving: 5

Keto Crepes

Buttery, delicious, and easy to make ahead and store!

½ C. coconut flour
4 Tb. coconut or vanilla sugar-free syrup
½ tsp. salt
6 eggs
¼ C. melted butter
¾ C. unsweetened coconut milk
1 tsp. vanilla extract
½ tsp. baking powder

Whisk together eggs, butter, coconut milk, vanilla extract, sugar-free syrup, and salt. In a separate bowl, combine coconut flour and baking powder. Mix wet and dry ingredients and allow the mixture to rest for about ten minutes to completely absorb. Heat a well-greased skillet to medium heat. Pour about ⅓ cup of the batter into the pan, swirling to coat the bottom of the skillet with a thin layer. When tiny bubbles appear, flip the crepe and cook until golden. Serve with sugar-free maple syrup, sugar-free jam, whipped cream, and fresh berries.

Servings: 4 (2 crepes each)

Net carbs per serving: 3

Keto Yogurt/Cereal

This granola recipe is crunchy (I can never get enough crunchy stuff on keto, since cereal is out!) and easy. It takes about ten minutes to make and is so yummy with coconut milk and berries!

1 C. almonds
1 C. pecans
1 C. hazelnuts
⅓ C. sunflower seeds
⅓ C. pumpkin seeds
½ C. ground flax seed
5 T. sugar-free vanilla syrup
1 egg white
¼ C. butter
¼ tsp. salt

Heat oven to 350 and prepare a baking sheet lined with parchment paper. While oven preheats, use a food processor to pulse the almonds and pecans into small chunks. Pour mixture into a bowl and set aside. Pulse pecans next, leaving chunks a bit larger. Add pecan chunks to nut mixture then add sunflower seeds, pumpkin seeds, and flax. In a separate bowl, whisk together the egg white, butter, syrup, and salt. Pour liquid mixture over the nut mixture and stir until well-coated. Pour granola onto the baking sheet in a thin, even layer and press into parchment with your hands. Bake for 15 minutes, then allow it to cool (it'll get crispy as it cools!).

Serving size: ¼ cup

Net carbs per serving: 2

Keto Cinnamon Breakfast Bread Pudding

This delicious bread pudding brings me back from the edge if I'm craving bready carbs. It's warm, yummy, and just so dang satisfying. Do NOT eat more than one serving at a time. This bread is PACKED with fiber, and it takes a second to register how full you are.

6 slices Franz Keto Bread, cut into 1-inch cubes
1.5 C. unsweetened coconut milk
1 Tb. cinnamon
¼ tsp. salt
4 Tb. melted butter
3 eggs
4 Tb. sugar-free vanilla syrup

Preheat oven to 375. Combine coconut milk and melted butter, then pour over bread chunks in a bowl. Let that mixture sit for about ten minutes. Meanwhile, mix eggs, cinnamon, salt, and vanilla syrup in a separate bowl. Pour egg mix over the bread and make sure all pieces are completely coated and saturated. Spoon the bread cubes into a greased baking pan, smooshing everything down so that the bread pieces are as close together as possible. Bake for 25 minutes. Serve with whipped cream, berries, low-carb chocolate chips, or sugar-free maple syrup.

Servings: 4

Net carbs per serving: 3.5

Keto Chorizo Scramble

5 eggs (beaten well)
3 oz. chorizo sausage (make sure you pay attention to whether it's mild or spicy! I accidentally got the spicy once, and it was a very sad morning).
½ C. cheddar cheese
4 Tb. green onion

Cook chorizo in a skillet until crumbled and browned. Turn heat down to low and add eggs and cheese. Don't rush this part. Let the eggs and cheese cook nice and slow, stirring once in a while, for about five minutes. Then garnish with the onions, and YUM!

Servings: 2

Net carbs per serving: 2

Super Easy, Low-Prep Breakfasts

The recipes above take less than half an hour to make. But some mornings, we don't have half an hour. I get it. So, in that spirit, I tend to make a lot of these recipes in bulk, so I have just ONE day of breakfast prep for the week. Or I rely on some of these go-to super-quick options:

- Hard-boiled eggs (about .5 net carbs each)
- Plain full-fat yogurt with stevia and sliced strawberries (½ cup of Fage total plain yogurt has 3.5 net carbs)
- Justin's Peanut butter squeeze packs (6 net carbs)
- Stoka or Kind Bars (Most Stoka bars are very low in net carbs, but you'll need to be choosier about the Kind bars. The nut-based options are your best bet).
- Low-carb protein shakes (I prefer the Isopure brand). Many are less than 3 net carbs per serving.
- A handful of almonds (just watch your portions). The carbs can add up, and you don't need that many nuts to feel full. ¼ cup of almonds has about 4.5 net carbs.

I hope these recipes give you a good jumping-off point to see the possibilities of keto breakfasts. If you crave it, you can find a recipe that's pretty darn close to what you're after—whether that's bread pudding, a smoothie, granola, eggs, a casserole: You name it. Make your breakfasts in bulk where possible, and experiment with your own substitutions and spices!

CHAPTER 9
Easy Lunches
That Legitimately Taste Good

I'll tell you right up front: I HATE lunch. I don't hate the food. I just hate making it. Because it's inevitably very inconvenient, and I just want something delicious that requires ZERO prep. So, you'll notice that all of the following recipes are VERY quick and easy. But they all legitimately taste delicious. If you want something fancier, move right along to the dinner recipes (and by "fancier" I mean that it'll take you twenty or thirty minutes instead of five or ten).

BBQ Ranch Chicken Wrap

This versatile wrap can be changed up with different types of deli meat, keto-friendly sauces (like vinaigrettes and low-sugar sauces), and different types of cheese. I make different variations of it often!

> 1 Carb Balance Mission Tortilla or low-carb wrap
> 2 Tb. shredded mozzarella or cheddar
> 1 tsp. sugar-free BBQ sauce
> 1 Tb. ranch (the full-fat stuff, not the lite crap)
> ¼ C. shredded lettuce
> 2 TB diced tomatoes
> ½ C. deli roasted chicken, diced

Place the tortilla on a baking sheet. Preheat the oven to 375. Sprinkle the cheese on top of the tortilla, then add the chicken. Drizzle the BBQ sauce on top and bake for about 5-7 minutes (or until cheese is melted and chicken is warm). Top with tomatoes, lettuce, ranch, and enjoy!

Servings: 1

Net carbs: 6 (this will obviously vary a little depending on the wrap or sauce you choose).

Keto Chopped Salad

2 hard-boiled eggs (You can use leftovers from breakfast!)
2 slices of cooked bacon (More breakfast leftovers!)
1 C. lettuce, shredded
½ avocado
¼ C. diced tomatoes
2 Tb. full-fat ranch
1 Tb. crispy onions (You can leave these off if you want, but they're delicious)

Toss all ingredients and enjoy!

Servings: 1

Net carbs: 6.5 (5 without the onions)

Keto Grilled Cheese

2 slices Franz Keto Bread
¼ C. shredded cheddar cheese
2 tsp. full-fat mayo
Garlic salt

Coat the outside of both pieces of bread with a thin layer of mayo and sprinkle garlic salt on top. Add cheese between bread slices and cook on the stovetop on low (this bread burns a little more easily, so take it easy on the heat) for about 5-7 minutes until both sides are golden brown and the cheese is melty and delicious.

Servings: 1

Net carbs 2

Shrimp and Avocado Salad

I love this simple, easy salad SO much. I get the pre-prepped cocktail shrimp to make this one extra fast and easy, but prep and boil (or sauté) your own if you have the time!

1 avocado, pitted and diced
10 medium shrimp, cooked and diced
1 Tb. sugar-free balsamic vinaigrette salad dressing
2 Tb diced green onions
Salt and pepper to taste

Toss everything together and enjoy!

Servings: 1

Net carbs: 4

Grilled Chicken and Cabbage Plate Lunch

2 chicken thighs
2 Tb. low-carb teriyaki sauce (try Primal Kitchen)
1 C. shredded coleslaw/cabbage
2 Tb low-carb sesame-ginger vinaigrette (try Ken's)
1 Tb. butter
½ C. riced cauliflower (you can get this in the frozen foods section with the veggies!)

Brush chicken with teriyaki sauce and grill for about 7 minutes per side, until cooked through. While you are grilling chicken, sauté the riced cauliflower in the butter until it is tender and beginning to turn golden brown. Top cauliflower with shredded cabbage, sliced chicken, and vinaigrette.
I tend to triple this recipe and eat it all week! But even if you make just one serving, it's still very quick and satisfying!

Servings: 1

Net carbs: 5 (depending on your dressing and sauce choices)

Keto Personal Pepperoni Pizza

Are you understanding how much I love Mission's Carb Balance tortillas? They make a fantastic pizza crust in this recipe!

1 Mission Carb Balance Tortilla
2 Tb. spaghetti sauce (Or pizza sauce, I can't taste the difference!)
¼ C. shredded mozzarella
10 pepperonis

Place the tortilla on a greased baking sheet. Spread sauce on top, then sprinkle mozzarella and pepperonis. Bake at 375 for about ten minutes, or until cheese is melted and tortilla edges are crisp. Allow pizza to cool for a couple of minutes, then either slice it into fourths or roll it up and eat it like a pizza rollup!

Servings: 1

Net carbs: 5

Shrimp and Sausage Skillet

This is another one that's ideal to make in a big batch and eat all week long!

1 pound uncooked shrimp, thawed and deveined
1 lb. pork sausage, sliced into ½-inch pieces
1 zucchini, diced
1 yellow squash, diced
1 Tb. olive oil
1 tsp. garlic
1 tsp. dried minced onion
2 tsp. Cajun seasoning

Toss shrimp, sausage, and veggies with olive oil. Transfer to a skillet, top with spices, and cook for about 10 minutes. Yum!

Servings: 5

Net carbs per serving: 5.5

Low-Carb Egg Rolls

This one takes just a little longer to make, but I love it for lunch because it saves so well (and can be made ahead of time in a big batch).

1 pound ground pork
1 Tb. fresh grated ginger (or t tsp. dry ginger)
1 Tb. sesame oil
1 tsp. garlic powder
1 bag shredded coleslaw
¼ C. soy sauce
2 Tb. rice vinegar
1/2 tsp. stevia in the raw (more if you like it sweeter)
2 Tb. diced green onions

Brown pork in a frying pan. Meanwhile, whisk together vinegar, stevia, soy sauce, and green onions. Drain pork, then add sesame oil, ginger, and garlic. Stir for about 1 minute, then add coleslaw. Cook for another 5 minutes until cabbage starts to wilt. Then top with the soy sauce mix and enjoy!

Servings: 4

Net carbs per serving: 7

Portobello-Stuffed Burger

Portobello mushrooms are tasty, filling, and more than make up for lack of a limp bun. I tend to eat this with a fork and knife, but you could always go full-animal and eat it with your hands. It's juicy!

1 portobello cap, stem removed
¼ lb. burger patty
2 Tb. shredded cheddar
1 tsp. minced onion
Shredded lettuce
4 pickles
1 slice tomato
Mustard and mayo

Fire up your grill (or set your oven to high broil). Spray or brush the portobello cap with oil and sprinkle with just a little salt. Season your burger as desired, and grill up the burger and portobello until tender and until the burger is no longer pink (about 5 minutes per side, for each). In the last few minutes of cooking, top both the burger and the portobello with half the cheese. Stack the burger on top of the portobello cap, then top with remaining condiments and enjoy!

Servings: 1

Net carbs: 4

Cheesy Taco Rolls

Make extra seasoned ground beef (that's the biggest time-suck on this recipe) and eat these for lunch all week!

3 oz. ground beef
2 tsp. taco seasoning
Salt and pepper to taste
½ C. cheddar cheese
Shredded lettuce
2 tsp. sour cream
Green salsa

On a piece of parchment paper, create two, street-taco-sized circles of shredded cheddar (just thick enough so you can't see parchment paper beneath the individual shreds). Bake the cheese at 375 degrees for around 10 minutes or until the cheese is totally melted and is just starting to turn golden (but isn't super brown or crispy yet). Meanwhile, brown up the ground beef. Allow the cheese circles to cool while you chop up the veggies. Then top each cheese circle with half of the ground beef, lettuce, sour cream, and green salsa. Roll up and enjoy!

Servings: 1

Net carbs: 5.5

Super Easy, Low-Prep Lunches

I rely on frozen meals for my low-prep lunches when I need to grab something FAST that will make me feel full and happy. There are a lot of frozen lunch options for low-carb available, and the variety will only increase as keto continues to grow in popularity.

My favorite frozen options are as follows:

- Atkins meals. Really all the varieties. Some of them look sort of "meh" on the box, but they are all pretty fresh and tasty.
- Performance kitchen: They are harder to find, but I love them! They're "small batch" and don't have the sad, mass-produced blob feel of a lot of frozen meals.
- Realgood Foods: Solid options, no preservatives. I loved pretty much all of their keto meals.

CHAPTER 10
Easy Dinners
That Legitimately Taste Good

You'll notice there are fewer lunches included in this book than dinners. Partly because, as we know, lunch annoys me as a concept. And partly because almost ALL of the following dinners can be saved as leftovers and eaten for lunch with basically NO prep.

As always, these keto dinner recipes are tried and tested, tasty, low-carb, and pretty darn easy. Also, they don't include any weird ingredients.

Keto Chicken Parmesan

8 boneless, skinless chicken thighs

¼ C. spaghetti sauce (I use Hunts, since it's on the lower end of the carb spectrum. Just be aware that some brands add a LOT of sugar, so keep an eye out.)

2 pieces Franz Keto Bread, well-toasted and crumbled in a food processor

½ tsp. garlic powder

¼ tsp. salt

½ tsp. dried parsley

1 C. mozzarella

2 zucchinis, cut into ½-inch rounds

1 tsp. olive oil

4 Tb. fresh basil, rough chopped (optional)

Brush chicken thighs with half the olive oil. Sprinkle with garlic powder and salt. Then press into the breadcrumbs and parsley (I put the breadcrumbs and parsley on a plate to do this, then press the thighs into them until a decent amount sticks). Place the thighs in a greased baking dish and bake at 375 for about 30 minutes. Remove from oven and drizzle with the spaghetti sauce. Then top with mozzarella and chopped basil. Bake for an additional 10 minutes.

While the chicken bakes, brush zucchini with remaining oil, sprinkle with salt and pepper, and sauté on medium high for five minutes on each side. Serve chicken over zucchini rounds, and save the leftovers for lunches!

Servings: 4

Net carbs per serving: 3.5

Artichoke Chicken

This one sounded weird to me until I actually tried it. I know it looks simple, but it's GOOD. The flavors meld so well, and it's such a tangy, tasty dish!

8 boneless, skinless chicken thighs
1 can artichoke hearts, drained and chopped
¾ C. parmesan cheese
1 Tb. Sundried tomatoes, finely minced
¾ C. mayo

Combine mayo, parmesan, artichoke hearts, and sundried tomatoes. Place chicken thighs in a greased baking dish. Cover chicken with mayo mixture, then bake at 375 for 35 minutes. Enjoy with low-carb veggies (like broccoli or Brussels sprouts).

Servings: 4

Net carbs per serving: 4

Candied Bacon-Wrapped Shrimp and Asparagus

10 large uncooked shrimp, thawed and deveined
4 pieces bacon, uncooked

10 spears of asparagus, washed and trimmed
Olive oil spray
Salt and pepper
1 Tb. sugar-free maple syrup

Servings: 1

Net carbs: 4.5

Preheat oven to 400. Spray asparagus and shrimp with olive oil, then sprinkle with salt and pepper. Divide asparagus into two bundles of five spears. Then wrap each bundle in a strip of bacon. Cut remaining two pieces of bacon into 5 even chunks each. Wrap and secure each chunk to a piece of shrimp with a toothpick. Place everything in a sprayed baking dish and drizzle with maple syrup. Bake for 10-12 minutes, until asparagus is tender, shrimp is opaque, and bacon is sizzling and browned.

One-Pan Buffalo Cauliflower and Steak

1/4 head cauliflower, sliced lengthwise into 1-inch steaks
3-oz tenderloin steak
½ C. parmesan, grated
2 Tb. full fat ranch dressing
1 tsp. Frank's red hot sauce
1 tsp. garlic salt
1 tsp. olive oil

Preheat oven to low broil. Prepare a rimmed baking sheet with parchment paper. Coat both sides of cauliflower and tenderloin with olive oil, then sprinkle with garlic salt. Sprinkle parmesan cheese on baking sheet in the shape of the cauliflower steaks, then place the cauliflower steaks on top of the parmesan. Place tenderloin next to the cauliflower on the parchment paper. Broil on low for 20 minutes, flipping steak once midway through. Drizzle ranch and Frank's on top of cauliflower and enjoy!

Servings: 1
Net carbs: 7

Shrimp Shirataki Scampi

Shirataki noodles are magic. They're a fantastic low-carb alternative to pasta, and they taste almost like full-carb noodles with the right sauce.

6 oz. shirataki noodles (spaghetti style)
20 thawed, uncooked, deveined shrimp
2 Roma tomatoes, diced
1 tsp. garlic powder
4 Tb. butter
2 Tb. lemon juice
1 tsp Worcestershire sauce
4 Tb. green onions
Salt and pepper to taste

Melt butter in a large skillet. Add green onions and garlic powder and stir for about 4 minutes. Add Worcestershire sauce, lemon juice, tomatoes, and shrimp. Cook until shrimp is just pink on both sides. Then add shirataki noodles. Stir well, and remove from heat for a few minutes for shirataki noodles to absorb sauce.

Servings: 2

Net carbs per serving 7

Deluxe Keto Burger

You can always make this one with a lettuce wrap, but the Franz Keto Buns are AMAZING. And they're just one carb each. (And super filling!) Make this recipe even easier with a frozen burger!

1 Franz Keto Hamburger Bun
½ tsp melted butter
¼ lb. raw ground beef
½ tsp. dried minced onion
½ tsp. Worcestershire sauce
⅛ tsp. salt
⅛ tsp. pepper
¼ C. cheddar cheese

¼ C. sliced mushrooms
Olive oil spray
Optional toppings: lettuce, tomato, pickles, mayo, mustard

Hand-mix ground beef with minced onion, Worcestershire sauce, salt, and pepper. Form into two patties, and grill for about 5 minutes on each side/until burgers are no longer pink in the center. Meanwhile, spray mushrooms with olive oil, sprinkle with salt, and grill them next to your burgers on a sheet of tin foil. Brush melted butter on the hamburger buns and lightly toast them on the grill. Top your burgers with the cheddar cheese in the last minute of cooking. Top your deluxe keto burger with lettuce, tomato, pickles, mustard, and mayo!

Servings: 1

Net carbs per serving: 2.5 (without optional toppings).

Deluxe Keto Dawg

SURPRISE! Franz makes a keto hot dog bun, too! This recipe is delicious, easy, and perfect for an easy barbecue.

2 keto hot dog buns
2 bratwursts (or hot dogs. Whatever you prefer. I really like the original Johnsonville brats)
4 Tb. sauerkraut
1 pickle, sliced thinly lengthwise
1 Tb. onion, chopped
1 tsp. mustard
1 tsp. Sugar-free Polynesian dipping sauce (G. Hughes brand, or use any other sweet and tangy low-carb sauce).

Make slices every inch or so along the brat or hot dog so that the smokiest flavor from the grill can be infused. Then grill the dog for about 7 minutes. Toast the bun as well, if desired. Top with sauerkraut, pickles, chopped onion, mustard, and Polynesian dipping sauce.

Servings: 2

Net carbs per serving: 4.5

Crispy Keto Battered Fish, Chips, and Tartar Sauce

For fish and chips:
2 lbs. cod, thawed, rinsed, and patted dry
¼ C. plain protein powder
⅔ C. almond flour
½ tsp. garlic salt
2 eggs
1.5 tsp. baking powder
⅓ C. club soda
1 zucchini, sliced into ½-inch "fries" and patted dry

For tartar sauce:
Mix all ingredients together (one serving is 1 tablespoon):
½ C. mayo
1 Tb. lemon juice
1 large pickle, diced
1 tsp. dill
¼ tsp. garlic salt
⅛ tsp. pepper

Place fish pieces and zucchini pieces on a baking sheet and sprinkle with half the garlic salt. In a separate bowl, combine remaining salt, protein powder, almond flour, and baking powder. Slowly add sparkling water and eggs. Mix well and allow the ingredients to rest for about five minutes. Meanwhile, heat oil in a deep pan to medium high. Once oil has heated, dip the fish pieces and zucchini pieces into the batter, one at a time, then carefully lower them into the hot oil. Don't overcrowd the pan. Cook in small batches until everything is cooked. Each batch will need about 5 minutes of cook time, with one flip midway through. Once fish/ fries are golden and cooked through, remove with tongs and place on paper towels to remove excess oil.

Serve with tartar sauce and lemon!

Servings: 4

Net carbs per serving: 6.5

Keto Meatloaf and Cauliflower au Gratin

This dish is such yummy comfort food! I love meatloaf, and the almond flour in this recipe helps absorb all those tasty juices as well as breadcrumbs. And the cauliflower au gratin is SO tasty!

Meatloaf:
2 pounds ground beef (I recommend 80/20 for the best flavor)
1 egg
½ c. finely ground almond flour
½ C. parmesan cheese
1 tsp. dried minced onion
2 tsp. garlic salt
¼ tsp. black pepper

Meatloaf glaze:
1 Tb. mustard
3 Tb. unsweetened ketchup
1/4 tsp. granulated stevia (or a couple of the drops of the liquid stuff. Just a touch of sweetness to that ketchup)

Preheat oven to 350. Use your hands (I know, gross, but it's the best way for best results) to thoroughly combine all meatloaf ingredients until well mixed. Form into a loaf and place it on a foil-lined, rimmed baking sheet. (If you bake it in a loaf pan, the meatloaf edges won't be nice and crispy!) Combine glaze ingredients and brush over entire surface of the meatloaf. Then bake for 1 hour.

Au gratin:
1 large cauliflower, cut into small pieces
½ tsp. garlic salt
Olive oil spray
1 C. cream
2 oz. cream cheese
1 tsp. mustard

2 C. shredded cheddar

Boil the cauliflower pieces until fork-tender (7 min). Drain and dry with paper towels. Meanwhile, in a saucepan combine cream cheese, cream, and mustard until melted and smoothly mixed. Whisk in 1.5 C. of cheese and garlic salt until cheese is melted. Place cauliflower pieces in a greased baking pan, then cover with melted cheese. Top with remaining grated cheese and bake for 20 minutes at 375.

Servings: 8

Net carbs per serving (for a serving of meatloaf along with a serving of au gratin): 3

Tangy Keto Meatballs and Zoodles

1 lb. pork sausage
1 lb. ground beef
½ C. grated parmesan
2 large eggs
1.5 C. grated mozzarella
2 tsp. garlic salt
2 tsp. onion powder
1 tsp. Italian seasoning
1 C. marinara sauce (I like Hunt's)
2 zucchini, spiralized

Preheat your oven to 375. In a big bowl, combine the pork, beef, parmesan, half of the mozzarella, eggs, and spices. Mix ingredients well by hand, then form into about 20 large meatballs. (You can use a ¼-cup measuring cup.) Place meatballs on greased baking pan and bake for 30 minutes. Then remove from oven, drain juices, and spoon marinara sauce on top of meatballs. Sprinkle remaining mozzarella on top and bake an additional 7 minutes until cheese is melted. Serve over spiralized zucchini.

Servings: 4

Net carbs per serving: 8

Keto Sushi Bowl

I love a good California roll. This bowl tastes so similar, and I love eating it!

½ C. riced cauliflower (Get it frozen for extra ease, or just process some florets in your food processor.)
½ tsp. butter
1 Tb. seasoned rice vinegar
¼ tsp. salt
½ avocado, diced
10 uncooked, deveined shrimp
1 Tb. mayo
1 tsp. sriracha sauce
2 Tb. green onions, chopped finely
3 oz. crab meat, rough chopped (You can get this canned or fresh from crab legs if you're feeling fancy. Just don't use the imitation stuff because it's full of carbs.)
1 sheet nori (dried seaweed)
Soy sauce to taste
Optional: cucumbers and bean sprouts

Melt butter in a skillet and cook riced cauliflower until tender. Remove from heat and drizzle with the rice vinegar and a sprinkle of the salt. Add shrimp to the same pan, sprinkle with salt, and cook until pink and firm on both sides. Top rice with shrimp, avocado, green onions, crab, and crumbled sheet of nori. Mix mayo and sriracha together and drizzle on top along with a little soy sauce. Enjoy! And feel free to add some cucumbers or bean sprouts (both low carb) if you so desire!

Servings: 1

Net carbs: 4

Keto Fajita Bowls

2 boneless, skinless chicken thighs
2 Tb. taco or fajita seasoning
2 Tb. butter

1 red bell pepper, thinly sliced
1 small red onion, thinly sliced
¼ C. fresh cilantro, chopped
1 avocado, peeled and chopped
1 C. lettuce, chopped
1 tomato, diced
2 Tb. sour cream
4 Tb. green salsa
½ C. cheddar

Thinly slice chicken, sprinkle with salt and pepper, and cook with the butter in a skillet until nearly cooked through (about 5-7 minutes). Add bell pepper and onion along with the taco seasoning, and cook until veggies are crisp-tender. Top with cheddar and turn off heat. While cheddar melts, prepare the lettuce, tomato, and avocado in bowls. Top lettuce mix with chicken mix and garnish with sour cream and green salsa. SO YUMMY!

Servings: 2

Net carbs per serving: 7

The Best Keto Clam Chowder

6 slices of salt pork (You can also use bacon, but it'll compete with the flavor of the clams instead of enhancing it!)
1 red onion, finely diced
1 head fresh cauliflower, chopped into small florets (don't use frozen, it'll get watery)
1 Tb. garlic powder
1 C. clam juice
12 oz. can of chicken broth
1 Tb. fresh thyme (you can also use 1 tsp. dried)
2 oz. cream cheese
4 cans chopped clams with juices (you can use less, but I like it CLAMMY)
1.5 C. heavy cream
1 Tb. vinegar

Salt and pepper to taste

In a deep pot, cook the salt pork until it's crispy. When it's nice and golden brown, remove the pieces of salt pork and place on paper towels to cool. In the same pot, sauté the garlic powder, onion, and the cauliflower until tender. Add cream cheese to stock pot and stir until melted. Then stir in chicken broth, clam juice, and thyme. Boil on low for about 25 minutes and allow flavors to meld. Slowly stir in the cream and simmer, stirring constantly, for about 5 minutes. Add clams and crumbled salt pork, then season with salt and pepper as desired and cook for 3-5 more minutes. Your taste buds are gonna thank me.

Servings: 6

Net carbs per serving: 6

Keto "Potato" Salad and BBQ Ribs

What, you say? Potato salad? This one should actually be called cauliflower salad (that's why "potato" is in quotes), but here's the thing: It tastes JUST like the real thing once you mix in that yummy sauce. And the ribs with sugar-free BBQ sauce are BOMB.

"Potato" salad
1 large head cauliflower, chopped into small (½ inch) florets and boiled with 1 tsp. of salt until fork tender (The same tenderness as you'd like a boiled potato!)
3/4 C. mayo
2 dill pickles, finely minced
½ sweet pickle, finely minced
½ tsp. powdered Stevia (or 3 drops liquid stevia concentrate)
¼ C. dill pickle juice
½ tsp. black pepper
1 Tb. vinegar
1 tsp. garlic powder
½ tsp. garlic salt
4 Tb. mustard
6 hard-boiled eggs, peeled and chopped
2 Tb. red onion, finely chopped

1 tsp. dried dill

Paprika for garnish

Place boiled cauliflower florets and chopped eggs in a bowl. In a separate bowl, mix remaining ingredients. Pour over cauliflower and eggs, garnish with paprika, and voila! Get ready to enjoy. I recommend refrigerating for about 2 hours prior to eating for best results, but I can never stop myself from just diving in.

Servings: 6

Net carbs per serving: 5.5

BBQ ribs

1 rack pork or beef ribs (any style)

1 tsp. garlic salt

1 tsp chili powder

1 tsp onion powder

1 tsp paprika

½ tsp. oregano

¼ tsp. cayenne pepper

¼ tsp. black pepper

Sugar-free BBQ sauce (I like Stubbs brand, but there are lots of options) for dipping

Preheat the oven to 300. Rinse and pat dry ribs, then place on a large sheet of tin foil. Combine all spices (except bay leaf) well, and then sprinkle mixture over ribs well until all surfaces are entirely coated. Wrap ribs tightly in tinfoil. Put tin foil packet on a baking sheet and cook for 3.5 hours. Remove ribs from oven, open foil (carefully!), and broil on high for about 5 minutes. Cut ribs into sections and dip into sugar-free BBQ sauce!

Servings: 6

Net carbs per serving (without BBQ sauce, make sure you account for that): 1

Keto Shepherd's Pie

1 head of cauliflower, chopped into small (½ inch) florets and boiled with 1 tsp. of salt until fork tender (The same tenderness as you'd like a boiled potato!)

> 4 oz. cream cheese
> 4 Tb. cream
> 1 tsp. garlic salt
> ¼ tsp. pepper
> 1 C. cheddar cheese
> ½ small red onion, finely chopped
> 1 lb. ground beef
> ½ C. beef broth
> Salt
> 1 tsp. olive oil
> ½ tsp. garlic salt
> 1 carrot, finely diced
> 1 tsp. garlic powder
> 1 Tb. tomato paste

Drain boiled cauliflower well and mash with cream cheese, cream, and garlic salt and pepper until smooth. Set aside. In a large skillet, cook onions, carrots, garlic powder, and ½ tsp. garlic salt until veggies begin to tenderize. Then add tomato paste and ground beef and cook until beef is browned and crumbled. And beef broth and simmer for about five minutes. Transfer beef mixture to a deep, greased baking pan. Spoon cauliflower mash on top. Sprinkle with cheddar and bake for 30 minutes at 350.

Servings: 4

Net carbs per serving. 6.5

Maple Mustard Pork Tenderloin and Zucchini Fries

Maple mustard pork:

1 pork tenderloin
4 Tb. dijon mustard
½ tsp. garlic salt
¼ tsp. pepper
2 tsp. olive oil
¼ C. apple cider vinegar
4 Tb. sugar-free maple syrup
1/2 tsp. dried sage

Preheat oven to 400. Mix 1 tablespoon of the dijon mustard, garlic salt, and pepper. Brush over tenderloin, then heat oil in a skillet and sear the outside of the pork on medium high until browned on all sides (this should take just a few minutes). Place pork in a baking dish. Combine remaining ingredients and pour over pork. Cook for about 20 minutes, or until pork reaches internal temperature of 145. Slice, and serve with zucchini fries!

Servings: 4

Net carbs per serving: 5

Zucchini fries:
Pop these babies in the oven before you start your pork, and they'll be ready at about the same time!

2 zucchini
⅔ C. grated parmesan
1 egg
½ tsp. garlic powder

Preheat oven to 400. Grease a baking sheet. Cut the zucchini lengthwise (4 times per zucchini) then crosswise, to create "fries" (each one will yield about 16 fries). Grab two bowls. In one bowl, beat the egg. In the other, combine the parmesan cheese and garlic. Dip each zucchini fry into the egg to coat, then the parmesan to coat (shake off the egg on each fry first to avoid getting a bunch of egg in your parmesan). Bake fries for 25 minutes, flipping midway through. Then broil on low for 5 additional minutes for extra crisp! Serve with ranch, low-carb marinara, or the drippings from your maple mustard pork. Yum!

Servings: 4

Net carbs per serving: 3

Cheesy Broccoli Soup

This one is such delicious comfort food. I will often eat it with the CarbQuik biscuits in the "Keto Sausage and Gravy" breakfast recipe.

2 large heads broccoli, chopped up into bite-sized pieces
1 Tb. garlic powder
4 C. chicken broth
1 C. cream
3 C. cheddar
¼ tsp. black pepper

Add all ingredients except cheddar to a large cooking pot. Simmer on medium low for about 20 minutes until broccoli is tender. Reduce heat to low and add cheese, one small handful at a time. (If you dump it all in, everything gets clumpy. Let each handful melt before adding a new one.) Remove from heat as soon as all cheese is melted and serve. YUM!

Servings: 8

Net carbs per serving: 4

Keto Butter Chicken and Naan

I love Indian food. So much. This recipe for butter chicken and naan is one of my favorites. It's a little carbier than some of these other recipes, but that's okay to include some higher-carb items in your rotation. Remember, we're all about sustaining our way of eating.

Butter Chicken:
2 lbs. boneless, skinless chicken thighs, cut into bite-sized pieces
½ C. full fat yogurt
1 tsp. garlic salt
2 tsp. garam masala

½ tsp. ground ginger
½ tsp. chili powder

Mix yogurt and spices together in a bowl. Then coat chicken liberally with mixture and refrigerate for two hours (or overnight, if you have the time). Meanwhile, make the sauce:

½ C. butter
½ C. onion, finely minced
2 cans tomato sauce (14 oz.)
1 tsp. garlic salt
1.5 Tb. garam masala
½ C. cream
1 tsp. ground ginger
1 tsp. chili powder
4 Tb. chopped fresh cilantro

Melt the butter and sauté the onions in a large skillet until they have softened. Stir in garlic and cook for about 1 minute. Add remaining ingredients and stir well. Remove chicken from marinade (no need to wipe off the marinade, just pull out the pieces with a slotted spoon and leave the remaining marinade behind) and add to the sauce mixture in the skillet. Mix gently and simmer for about 10 minutes, stirring every few minutes until the chicken is fully cooked.

Servings: 6

Net carbs per serving: 8

Naan:
3 C. mozzarella
2 eggs
3 T. Greek yogurt (full fat)
2 tsp garlic powder, divided
1 ¼ C. almond flour
1 Tb. baking powder
2 Tb. melted butter
2 Tb. fresh chopped cilantro

Heat oven to 375. Mix Greek yogurt, 1 tsp. garlic powder, and mozzarella in a microwave-safe bowl and microwave for about 3 minutes, stirring every minute, until mixture is smooth. In a separate bowl, combine eggs, almond flour, and baking powder. Fold hot cheese mixture into almond flour mixture. You'll need to mix by hand, until you get a smooth, elastic dough. If dough is super sticky, just pop it into the fridge for about 10 minutes. Then divide dough into 6 sections, roll each section into a ball, and flatten/stretch it until it's about as thick as your pinky finger. Bake on parchment paper for 10 minutes. Combine melted butter, 1 tsp. garlic powder, and cilantro. Remove naan from oven, brush with butter, and return to oven for about 3 minutes.

Servings: 6

Net carbs per serving: 1

Garlic Butter Steak and Caprese

Caprese:
1 fresh tomato
2 Tb. fresh basil, chopped into ribbons
1 ball fresh mozzarella
1 Tb. olive oil
1 Tb. balsamic vinegar
Salt and pepper to taste

Slice tomato into 6 slices. Liberally salt and pepper each piece. Slice the mozzarella into 6 even slices and place each mozzarella slice on top of each tomato slice. Drizzle each piece with olive oil and balsamic vinegar, then sprinkle fresh basil over the top.

Garlic butter steak:
1 thick boneless ribeye (about 2 inches thick)
½ tsp. Garlic salt
¼ tsp. Pepper
1 Tb. vegetable oil
4 cloves garlic, minced
1 Tb. fresh rosemary, finely chopped

Season steak with salt and pepper on both sides. Place on rimmed baking sheet and cook for 1 hour in a 200-degree oven. Heat vegetable oil in a skillet until very hot (but not smoking). Sear steak for 30 seconds on each side, then add the garlic, butter, and rosemary to the pan. Flip steak to coat each side with butter mix, then remove from heat. All to rest for 5-7 minutes, then cut and enjoy!

Servings: 2

Net carbs per serving: 4.5 (this is for one serving of caprese plus one serving of steak)

CHAPTER 11
Easy Snacks
That Legitimately Taste Good

Fair warning: The recipes in this section are SUPER simple. Some aren't even recipes. They're just things you can buy and eat as snacks when you need one. If you're someone who LOVES making 30-minute snack recipes in the middle of your day in addition to other meals, there are loads of books out there that will make you happy. I personally hate those recipe books. Because I barely have time to cook meals, let alone snacks. So, that said, here are some VERY quick snack options that taste great:

Peanut Butter and Celery

This snack is satisfying, crunchy, and EASY. Just spread peanut butter onto the celery sticks and enjoy!

2 Tb. peanut butter
1 C. celery sticks (about 10 sticks)

Servings: 1

Net carbs: 3

Strawberries and Yogurt

½ C. full-fat, unsweetened yogurt (I use Fage, it's the lowest carb count I can find.)
3 packets stevia (Or more, depending on your sweetness preference. You can also use drops.)
½ tsp. vanilla extract

1/4 C. diced strawberries

Mix yogurt, stevia, and vanilla extract well. Then top with berries.

Servings: 1

Net carbs: 4.5

Nuts

Most nuts will do you right for a quick snack. Just make sure you measure your quantities (because it's easy to pop a TON of nuts in your mouth before you even realize you're full or have actually eaten a few too many carbs).

Here are the net carbs and servings of a few of the lowest-carb nuts:

¼ C. roasted Brazil nuts: 1 net carbs
¼ C. roasted walnuts: 2 net carbs
¼ C. roasted macadamia nuts: 2 net carbs
¼ C. roasted almonds: 3 net carbs
¼ C. roasted hazelnuts: 3 net carbs
¼ C. roasted pine nuts: 3 net carbs
¼ C. pistachios: 5 net carbs
¼ C. peanuts: 5 net carbs

Hard-Boiled Egg

This is as easy as it gets. Although I do like to mash mine up with a little melted butter, salt, and pepper! If you're feeling really wild, make yourself some quick deviled eggs. Both the butter and the mayo will add negligible carbs!

Net carbs in one hard-boiled egg: 1

Pork Rinds

There are ZERO net carbs in pork rinds! Woohoo! You can dip them in salsa, or just enjoy them out of the bag.

Net carbs: 0

Granola Bars

There are a number of very tasty, low-carb granola bars out there. Here are my top faves in terms of taste and carb count:

Kind Bar, Dark Chocolate Cherry Cashew: 8 net carbs
IQ Bar, Almond Butter Chip: 3 net carbs
Dang Bar, Lemon: 5 net carbs
Atlas Protein Bar, Chocolate: 3 net carbs
Keto Krisp, Almond Butter: 4 net carbs
Keto Bars, Dark Chocolate Coconut Almond: 3 net carbs

Celery and Ranch

2 Tb. ranch
1 C. celery sticks (about 10 sticks)

Servings: 1

Net carbs: 3

Protein Shake

A protein shake is a perfectly satisfying, hydrating pick-me-up on keto. I like the Isopure Dutch Chocolate, but there are lots of good ones. Just one gram of net carbs per serving!

Ham, Egg and Cheese Rolls

This snack takes a TAD more time, but it's so yummy! This also makes a good breakfast.

6 slices of ham
6 slices cheddar or pepper jack cheese
2 tsp. butter
2 T. chopped green onions

4 large eggs
Salt and pepper

Whisk eggs with green onions and a pinch of salt and pepper. Cook the eggs in the butter until JUST done. Place the cheese slices on top of the ham slices, the spoon a dollop of eggs on top of the cheese. Then roll each ham slice up tightly until you have a nice little tube. Place tubes side-by-side in a baking dish and bake for about 10 minutes on 375!

Servings: 6

Net carbs per serving: 1.5

Quesadilla and Salsa

1 Mission Carb Balance Tortilla
¼ C. shredded cheddar

Spray a skillet well, then toast one side of a tortilla for about 30 seconds on medium heat. Flip tortilla over, sprinkle cheese on one half, then fold over. Cook quesadilla on both sides until golden brown, and serve with your favorite low-carb salsa. (Green salsa is usually a very solid bet, but most salsas are quite low carb!)

Servings: 1

Net carbs: 4

Keto Chips and Guac

1 Mission Carb Balance Tortilla, sliced into eight triangles
1 tsp. oil
Salt
1/2 avocado
½ tsp. lime juice
¼ tsp. salt
¼ tsp. pepper
1 tsp. chopped onion

Preheat oven to 350. Place tortilla sections on parchment paper and brush both sides with oil, lightly. Then sprinkle with salt and bake for 5-7 minutes until chips are lightly golden and crunchy. Mix remaining ingredients for guacamole, and enjoy!

Servings: 1

Net carbs: 4

CHAPTER 12
Easy Desserts
That Legitimately Taste Good

Wait, we get to eat desserts? Yeah, you do. But I want to start this chapter with a teensy, weensy caveat: This chapter is especially important because a lot of keto desserts taste kind of horrible. You'll see this beautiful-looking piece of cake, you'll take a bite, and you'll think, "What the fresh hell was that?"

I learned this firsthand when I baked a keto cake for my husband's birthday. We had just started keto. We were doing it. We were feeling better and losing weight. But it was his birthday, so we both wanted a little treat that wouldn't mess with our new success. So I naively picked the first recipe for keto chocolate cake that I found on the Internet.

It looked good in the pictures. It looked good when I baked it. I was excited. My husband was excited. The kids were even excited. They took the first bites. And they literally SCREAMED and spit it out. I thought they were being dramatic, so I took a bite. And it was so bad. I can't even describe it to you.

I've learned a lot since then. The trick is to find REAL foods that taste great with a few tweaks. Trying to make a cake out of stevia and psyllium husk is risky business. Here's the (easy, tasty) desserts I've found that I go back to over and over again. By all means, scour the internet and try new stuff. You'll find some good ones. But READ THE REVIEWS and be wary of recipes that sound extra complex or rely on strange ingredients. Desserts are usually loaded with carbs. Because they're sweet. Stevia is great, but it can only get you so far. I hope you enjoy these treats as much as I do. But the truth is, I don't make them that often. And you won't either. Because keto is all about resetting your body and helping you withdraw from sugar addictions. And when you do that, you don't crave sweet things constantly.

Now to the desserts. Because sometimes they still do hit the spot!

Any-Flavor Mug Cake

Mug cakes are the best. They're easy, quick, and single serve. Plus, as you may have guessed from the title, you can easily make them any flavor with easy adjustments. I'll give you the base recipe first, then a list of ideas for flavors:

Mug cake base:
2 T. CarbQuik

1 T. melted butter

1 T. heavy cream

1 pinch salt

1 tsp granulated stevia (or you can use another no-sugar sweetener, or 5 drops of liquid stevia concentrate)

½ tsp. baking powder

1 egg, well beaten

½ tsp. vanilla

Melt butter in your mug. Allow it to cool slightly, then add remaining ingredients and mix well. Add your choice of ingredients below, then microwave for 60 seconds and enjoy with whipped cream or sugar-free chocolate chips.

Add-ins:
For chocolate: 1 Tb. unsweetened baking powder

For chocolate mint: 1 Tb. unsweetened baking powder, 1 Tb sugar-free peppermint syrup

For chocolate-peanut butter: 1 Tb. peanut butter + 1 Tb. unsweetened baking cocoa (melt the peanut butter with the butter for your first step!)

For blueberry: ¼ C. fresh or frozen blueberries

For lemon poppyseed: ½ tsp. poppyseeds and ½ tsp. lemon juice

Servings: 1

Net carbs per serving: 3-7, depending on which ingredients you choose

110

Chocolate Mascarpone Mousse

This dessert is extremely rich and extremely tasty. Savor it with berries, whipped cream, or sugar-free chocolate chips! If you prefer vanilla mousse, just leave out the chocolate.

4 oz. mascarpone
½ C. whipping cream
1 tsp. vanilla
1 Tb. unsweetened baking cocoa powder
1 tsp. sugar-free syrup (can be any flavor you like, but I use vanilla)

Mix all ingredients well using a hand mixer. Enjoy!

Servings: 6

Net carbs per serving: 1.5

Strawberry Ice Cream

This recipe is SO delicious and fresh!

2 C. fresh strawberries
1 C. monk fruit powder
2 C. cream
1 C. sour cream
1 tsp. vanilla extract
½ tsp. freshly squeezed lemon juice (It's worth it to use fresh!)

Use a blender or food processor to pulse strawberries, monk fruit powder, and vanilla until combined but still chunky. Let everything sit for at least half an hour (at room temp) to combine flavors. Otherwise, you're gonna get a weird aftertaste from the monk fruit sweetener.

Add sour cream, cream, and lemon juice. Pulse until the mixture is pretty smooth and very well combined. Pour everything into an ice cream maker and follow your machine's direction. If you don't have an ice cream maker, you can also pour everything into a glass pan and freeze for a couple of hours!

Servings: 8

Net carbs per serving: 6

Easy Keto Strawberry Sundae

If you don't have the energy to make ice cream from scratch, Breyer's Carb Balance is my favorite base for a sundae treat!

⅔ C. Breyer's Carb Balance Vanilla Ice Cream
Small handful of dark chocolate chips (about 2 Tb.)
¼ C. sliced strawberries
Whipped cream
Sugar-free chocolate sauce

Servings: 1

Net carbs: 6

Keto CarbQuik Cobbler

This recipe is SO tasty and satisfying. I love it for a fall day or while camping! (You can make it ahead and cook in a dutch oven if you like!)

2 C. frozen or fresh blackberries
¼ c. monk fruit powder
1 tsp. fresh lemon juice
4 Tb. butter, melted
1 tsp. cinnamon
1 C. CarbQuik
½ C. coconut milk
½ tsp. cornstarch
1 egg
1 tsp. vanilla
3 Tb. monk fruit powder

Combine blackberries, cornstarch, ¼ C. monk fruit powder, and lemon juice. Combine well and pour into a sprayed baking pan. Combine

CarbQuik, melted butter, 3 Tb. monk fruit powder, egg, cinnamon, vanilla, and coconut milk. Place spoonfuls of CarbQuik mixture evenly over berries. Bake for 20 minutes at 400 degrees, and serve with a drizzle of cream!

Servings: 6

Net carbs per serving: 6

Keto Cheesecake

This is the real deal. Plus it's easy—and saves great in the fridge!

Crust
2 C. finely ground almond flour
⅓ C. melted butter
1 tsp. cinnamon
3 T. monk fruit powder
2 tsp. vanilla extract

Filling
32 oz. softened cream cheese
3 large eggs
2 tsp. vanilla extract
1 tsp. fresh lemon juice
1 ¼ C. monk fruit powder

Grease a 9-inch round springform and preheat your oven to 350. Combine crust ingredients until well mixed and crumbly. Press into the bottom of the greased springform and bake for 10 minutes. While crust is cooling, beat cream cheese and monk fruit powder until fluffy. Then slowly beat in eggs, lemon juice, and vanilla. Pour filling on top of crust and bake for 50 minutes. It's okay if the cheesecake doesn't look totally set/is a little runny in the middle. Cool the cheesecake, then pop it into the fridge overnight (or for a few hours at least) and enjoy! Top it with whipped cream, blueberries, raspberries, or strawberries!

Servings: 16

Red Velvet Fat Bombs

These little babies are incredibly good and so easy. I love having them on hand for a quick fix! And you can easily freeze them to save for a rainy day.

4 oz. 90% cacao chocolate
4 oz. cream cheese, softened to room temp
3 Tb. monk fruit powder
4 oz. unsalted butter, softened to room temp
6 drops red food coloring
2 tsp. vanilla extract

Microwave chocolate, 30 seconds at a time and stirring at each interval, until melted and smooth. In a separate bowl, use a hand mixer to combine all other ingredients. Then slowly add in chocolate. Spread parchment paper on a cookie sheet and plop heaping spoonfuls of mixture (it should yield about 24 heaping spoonfuls) onto the parchment. Refrigerate for about an hour and enjoy! These keep well in the fridge for at least a week and can be saved in the freezer for much longer.

Servings: 24

Net carbs per serving: 1

Fudgy Brownies

My kids will eat these without complaint. Which is really saying something. We've come a long way.

1 C. finely ground almond flour
⅓ C. baking cocoa powder
1 tsp. baking powder
⅓ C. melted butter
¼ tsp. salt
⅓ C. melted butter

2 eggs
⅔ C. monk fruit powder
2 tsp. vanilla extract
2 Tb. water

Preheat your oven to 350. Mix all ingredients until batter is smooth. Bake in a greased 8-inch baking pan for 25 minutes. I love eating these with Carb Balance vanilla ice cream!

Servings: 15

Net carbs per serving: 2

CHAPTER 13
Eating Out on Keto

This section deserves its own chapter. Because, if you're anything like me, you love eating out. Cooking can be hard on the best days. And it's just so satisfying to have someone else make you a meal.

General Advice for Eating Out

The happy truth is, you can find something tasty and keto-friendly at almost any restaurant. But it can be really helpful to have a general idea of go-to options on the menu, since it's not always feasible or even possible to aggressively consult your phone on carb counts.

When you eat out, your goal is a win-win: Something that tastes good AND keeps you in ketosis. Yes, there will be times when you decide to "cheat" and go full carb. But make that experience the exception rather than the rule. Because you'll be pleasantly surprised how many tasty options you can find at chain- and non-chain restaurants.

My Favorite Go-Tos at Almost Any Restaurant

You can find keto go-to's at almost any restaurant. And if you can't? Well, then it's time to get creative with the substitutions.

If you can't find low-carb entrees, make a meal out of low-carb apps. Ask for celery sticks instead of chips with that guacamole. Look for protein-centric meals. Sub a bun for lettuce. Swap the mashed potatoes for sauteed veggies. Most places will be more than happy to accommodate you.

I like to try to look at the menu ahead of time, but I've learned to watch out for particular kinds of foods at different restaurants. Here's what I seek out as solid keto options at different types of restaurants:

Japanese: Sashimi, miso soup, seaweed salad, and hibachi items are typically very safe bets. Just skip the rice!

Burger joint: This one can be tough, but I like to skip the bun in favor of lettuce and add in a lot of extras like bacon, avocado, and mushrooms to make up for the loss! Zucchini fries are a great option for sides, as long as they're not heavily breaded.

Pizza place: Another tough one. But more and more places are offering cauliflower crust. (Like Blaze Pizza!) If no keto-friendly crusts are available, look for wings on the apps menu, ask for a small pizza with extra cheese and lots of tasty toppings—and just eat the top half of the pizza without the crust! Some chains even offer "pizza bowls" with lots of toppings and cheesy goodness.

Steakhouse: Finally, an easy bet! Steak is a great keto choice. Pair it with sauteed veggies instead of a baked potato and enjoy a salad with some full-fat or oil-based dressing.

Seafood restaurant: Another winner with lots of options. Most seafood is keto-friendly as long as it isn't fried and battered. Enjoy seafood like salmon, clams, crab, lobster, cod, you name it! Just don't pair it with fries!

Chinese: Look for non-breaded, non-noodly items without a lot of sweet sauces. Some good options include kung pao chicken, chicken and snow peas, Peking duck, egg drop soup, beef and broccoli, and other sauteed proteins with veggies!

Indian: Skip the naan and rice, but you can typically enjoy butter chicken, tandoori chicken, kormas, and other main dishes with curries and creamy sauces! I like to order something veggie-heavy and something sauce-based, then top the veggies with sauce!

Mexican: While you'll want to stay away from taco shells or rice and beans, there are some excellent options available in most Mexican restaurants. Fajitas are a fantastic choice, as well as most taco salads. (Again, just skip the rice and beans!) Guacamole is a great choice, and

I'll often order fajitas sans tortillas, loaded up with sour cream, extra cheese, and guac!

Popular Chain Options

Restaurants are all well and good, but what about when you're in the car and feeling low on fuel? These quick-fix chain options are available in most states, and all of them have good keto options on the menu:

Starbucks: The Creminelli Sopressata Monterey Jack Snack Tray is basically a mini charcuterie board. And the sous vide gruyere and bacon bites are fabulous (the mushroom ones are pretty good too)! For coffee, I recommend ordering a basic iced or hot Americano with an extra splash of heavy cream (it makes it SO creamy!) and sugar-free syrup flavoring. It tastes just like a latte!

McDonald's: If you need a tasty (and cheap) breakfast sandwich, this is the place to go. You can typically get two sausage egg and cheese breakfast sandwiches for a solid deal (right now it's $4), sans bun. Burgers and grilled chicken sandwiches sans bun are solid lunch options as well.

Wendy's: This is my favorite place to enjoy a lettuce wrap burger. The burgers are a generous size, nobody has ever blinked twice when I order sans bun, and the meat is fresh instead of frozen. I'll typically get a Dave's double with cheese, no bun. It's surprisingly filling! Wendy's chicken sandwiches are pretty darn tasty as well. (No bun!)

Blaze Pizza: The keto crust option is SO good. It's made from mozzarella, cauliflower, and flax. Top it with red sauce, mozzarella, and any of your favorite toppings (I personally LOAD it to the max with all the meats and veggies). Each slice ends up being about 2 net carbs! And it'll fill you up, with so much fiber.

Olive Garden: Plenty of options here. (Just say no to the breadsticks!) The herb-grilled salmon, chicken piccata, and the salad (without croutons) are all good bets. Opt for the parmesan-garlic broccoli for a solid keto side!

Chipotle: Bless Chipotle: they recently introduced cauliflower rice to their menu, so you don't even have to skip the rice! Choose a bowl rather than a burrito, since the tortilla packs a big carb punch. My ideal bowl is cauliflower rice with grilled chicken (steak is another good choice, but it's too spicy for my tastes), pico, guac, sour cream, cheese, sauteed veggies, and lettuce.

Buffalo Wild Wings: Honestly, this is one of my favorite places to eat out on Keto. There's just something so juicy and indulgent about eating wings with your hands! Make sure you choose the original wings (not the boneless) and opt for a non-carby sauce. The parmesan garlic and original buffalo sauces are safe bets. And you can choose any of the dry rubs. (BBQ and salt and vinegar are my favorite dry rubs!) Ask for lots of celery and ranch to accompany your wings, and you've got a delicious keto treat.

Outback: Outback has tons of good keto options. Any of the steaks, the lobster tail, shrimp, and almost any salmon or fish option are good choices. Add sauteed mushrooms and broccoli or asparagus to round out your meal!

Jack in the Box: Similar to Wendy's and McDonald's, just order a bunless burger here. I love the Double Jack! Like Wendy's, the burger patty at Jack in the Box is substantial, well-seasoned, and satisfying. The grilled chicken sandwiches are also safe keto bets, when bunless.

Taco Bell: The Taco Bell Power Bowl with chicken or steak—minus the beans and rice, sub in extra chicken and guac—is my go-to here. It makes a pretty filling, pretty tasty meal on the go!

Panda Express

My favorites at Panda include the grilled teriyaki chicken (just skip the sauce or go SUPER light with it), the broccoli beef, black pepper Angus steak, mushroom chicken, and string bean chicken breast. All of them are tasty and satisfying. I'll often add an extra side of broccoli to enjoy with my meal.

Panera: All of Panera's breakfast wraps are pretty tasty (sans wrap) on keto. You can also make a lettuce wrap out of their sandwiches, like the roasted turkey and avocado BLT or the chipotle chicken avocado melt. Be wary of the salads (lots of them pack a wallop with carbs). The Caesar salad, sans croutons, is a good option. And the Greek salad with light onions and tomatoes is a good bet.

KFC: Definitely avoid the breaded chicken at KFC, but the grilled chicken has less than 1 gram of net carbs! Steer clear of the mashed potatoes and opt for green beans as a side.

Arby's: Almost any sandwich at Arby's can be served in a bowl. Enjoy a classic roast beef, a Beef 'N Cheddar, french dip, etc. Just skip any red sauce, honey mustard, or other sweet sauces like barbecue. Arby's sauce, red ranch sauce, horsey sauce, cheese sauce, and mayo can all be added! Salads without croutons are pretty good here too, with some bacon and ranch or Italian dressing.

That's my playbook for eating out. That said, I do try to make most of my meals at home. It's easier to avoid unexpected carbs in sauces, etc. that way. Not to mention that portions can sometimes be harder to guess, and fast food just tends to be carbier in general. It's also easier to resist the temptation of adding a Frosty to my meal, "just this once!"

However, I've found that when I follow these guidelines for eating out, I can stay in ketosis and keep my goals!

CHAPTER 14
Two-Week Meal Plan and Shopping List

You've got your recipes. And you've got your go-to options for the times you don't really feel like cooking. But sometimes, it really helps to have a clear plan moving forward. That's why I've included this chapter with a two-week meal plan.

I'm including a breakfast, lunch, dinner, and snack for each day, with a couple of desserts included in the week for you to look forward to. I've also included your total net carbs per day, so you'll know whether you have some wiggle room. Remember: You don't need to go hungry. That never feels good. If you're hungry and you're out of carbs, you've got options. (Just get back to that snacks chapter!)

This two-week meal plan is just a starting point. If you want to follow it exactly, great! If not, mix and match recipes as you see fit. You'll notice that I've given you carbs to spare each day, so you can add low-carb beverages and side-dishes (like non-starchy veggies, side salads, etc.) to your meals. You can also add in a little extra treat each day if you so desire, like some dark chocolate (just watch those portions).

I know some people love their side dishes for meals. I personally prefer to keep it simple and add some steamed broccoli with my main dish once in a while. If you love sides, there are plenty of options to be found in the recipe chapters!

Shopping List

Make sure you consult the recipes in Week 1 and Week 2 first before you grab up all these groceries. If you want to substitute any recipes, just make sure you add and delete shopping list items accordingly! Also, this shopping list is for one person. If you're shopping for two people, double list items and recipes accordingly!

One last note on this shopping list: You'll already have heavy cream and stevia on this list, so you can make a plentitude of coffee drinks with those alone. Add carbonated seltzers, herbal teas, and other beverages to your shopping list as you so desire!

Dairy
2 dozen eggs

1 quart half-and-half

1 pint heavy cream

4 sticks of salted butter

1 package full-fat sour cream

1 container (needs to contain 1 C. total) full-fat plain yogurt without added sugar

1 large package shredded cheddar cheese

1 large package shredded mozzarella cheese

1 package shredded parmesan

1 container of full-fat ranch dressing (Litehouse brand is great!)

6 oz. cream cheese, full fat

1 ball fresh mozzarella

4 oz. mascarpone

Meat
1 pound Jimmy Dean pork sausage

1 pound ground pork

1 package mild chorizo sausage (or go spicy, if you like!)

1 family pack of boneless, skinless chicken thighs (make sure you get 16 thighs)

30 large shrimp (fresh or frozen)

1 package bacon

3-oz. tenderloin steak

3-oz. fresh crab meat (can be canned or from crab legs, just don't use the imitation stuff)

2 pounds ground beef

1 package pepperoni (or other pizza topping)

1 package uncured salt pork

1 thick, boneless ribeye steak

Spices and Condiments
(You'll likely already have many of these but including them here so you know!)

Garlic powder
Garlic salt
Fresh or dried thyme
Fresh or dried ginger
Sesame oil
Salt
Apple cider vinegar
Balsamic vinegar
Powdered stevia
Monk fruit powder
Pepper
Parsley
Taco seasoning
Frank's hot sauce
1 bottle full-fat mayo
Rice vinegar
Sriracha sauce
Soy sauce
Lemon juice
Dried, minced onions
Worcestershire sauce
Pickles
*Optional: Additional low-carb burger condiments like mustard

Canned Food
Green salsa
1 jar spaghetti sauce (I use Hunt's four-cheese; choose the lowest carb count you can!)
1 bottle clam juice
1 12-oz. can chicken broth
4 cans chopped clams
1 can artichoke hearts
1 jar sun-dried tomatoes

Frozen Foods

1 package riced cauliflower
1 container Breyer's Carb Balance Vanilla Ice Cream

Fresh Produce

1 bundle of green onions
1 portobello cap
1 pint strawberries
2 zucchinis
1 bunch fresh basil
1 bunch asparagus
2 heads of cauliflower
2 avocados
4 Roma tomatoes (More if you want them for your burgers!)
1 head lettuce
1 package fresh, sliced mushrooms
2 small red onions
1 head of garlic
Fresh rosemary
Celery
1 bag shredded coleslaw

Pantry

(Again, you probably have a lot of these already, but I'm being thorough!)

1 package CarbQuik (You may need to get this via Amazon.)
Shirataki noodles (You can usually find these in the Asian or international section.)
Dark chocolate chips
Cooking spray
Low-carb chocolate protein powder (or whatever flavor you prefer)
1 bottle extra-virgin olive oil
1 bottle sugar-free maple syrup
1 small package nori sheets
1 jar peanut butter
Roasted, salted almonds
Baking powder

Vanilla sugar-free flavored syrup for mug cakes, mousse, and beverages

4 oz. 90% cacao chocolate

Baking cocoa

Vanilla extract

Crispy onions

Pork rinds

Baked Goods

1 package Mission Carb Balance Tortillas

1 package Franz Keto bread

1 package Franz Keto hamburger buns

Week 1

Week 1 is the hardest. Which is why I've packed this week with my MOST delicious, most favorite recipes to ease you in. You're still going to have to battle some carb withdrawals. It happens. But it won't last, and in the meantime you can enjoy lots of delicious food. Be extra kind to yourself this week, and don't try to plan anything crazy.

You'll notice that I started the week off on Sunday, and I recommend you do the same. Why? Because this gives you time to spend a little more energy making meals that will last with leftovers. If you work on Sundays or this is a busy day for you, start your week on whatever day is least busy for you. And again, this meal plan is only a guide. If you want to spend more time in the kitchen or making different recipes, do it!

Sunday

Breakfast

Keto chocolate chip waffles/pancakes: 2 pancakes (Refrigerate two more for Monday's breakfast, and freeze the remainder for next week.)

Net carbs: 4

Lunch

Keto Personal Pepperoni Pizza

Net carbs: 5

Dinner
Keto Chicken Parmesan: 1 serving (Save the remaining 3 servings for lunches! Easy!)
Net carbs: 3.5

Snack
2 Tb peanut butter and 10 sticks celery
Net carbs: 3

Dessert
Any-Flavor Mug Cake, 1 serving
Net carbs: 4 (depending on add-ins)

Total daily net carbs: 19.5

Monday

Breakfast
Leftover Keto chocolate chip waffles/pancakes: 2 pancakes
Net carbs: 4

Lunch
Leftover Keto Chicken Parmesan: 1 serving
Net carbs: 3.5

Dinner
Candied Bacon-Wrapped Shrimp and Asparagus
Net carbs: 4.5

Snack
¼ C. roasted, salted almonds
Net carbs: 3

Total daily net carbs: 15

Tuesday

Breakfast
Keto Salsa Verde Breakfast Burrito: 1 burrito
Net carbs: 6

Lunch
Leftover Keto Chicken Parmesan: 1 serving
Net carbs: 3.5

Dinner
One-Pan Buffalo Cauliflower and Steak
Net carbs: 7

Snack
Quesadilla and salsa, 1 serving
Net carbs: 4

Total daily net carbs: 20.5

Wednesday

Breakfast
½ C. yogurt with stevia topped with ¼ C. sliced strawberries
Net carbs: 4.5

Lunch
Leftover Keto Chicken Parmesan: 1 serving
Net carbs: 3.5

Dinner
Shrimp Shirataki Scampi: 1 serving (Save your other serving for lunch tomorrow!)
Net carbs: 2

Snack
2 Tb peanut butter and 10 sticks celery
Net carbs: 3

Dessert
Easy Keto Strawberry Sundae, 1 serving
Net carbs: 6

Total daily net carbs: 19

Thursday

Breakfast

Keto Chorizo Scramble: 1 serving (Save the other serving in the fridge for tomorrow!)
Net carbs: 2

Lunch

Leftover Shrimp Shirataki Scampi
Net carbs: 2

Dinner

Deluxe Keto Burger
Net carbs: 2.5

Snack

2 Tb peanut butter and 10 sticks celery
Net carbs: 3

Total daily net carbs: 9.5

Friday

Breakfast

Leftover Keto Chorizo Scramble: 1 serving
Net carbs: 2

Lunch

Keto Grilled Cheese, 1 serving
Net carbs: 2

Dinner

Keto Sushi Bowl
Net carbs: 4

Snack

1 serving chocolate protein shake
Net carbs: 3 (Your brand might be lower!)

Dessert

Red Velvet Fat Bomb, 2 servings (Freeze the rest, we'll eat them as treats in Week 2!)
Net carbs: 2

Total daily net carbs: 13

Saturday

Breakfast
1 serving of Keto Biscuits and Gravy (Refrigerate the remaining 2 servings of sauce and biscuits for Week 2, and freeze the rest for another week!)
Net carbs: 7

Lunch
Cheesy Taco Rolls
Net carbs: 5.5

Dinner
Keto clam chowder: 1 serving (This is a little bit time-intensive, but it's SO good for leftovers and is going to provide easy lunches for most of next week!)
Net carbs: 6

Snack
2 Tb ranch and 10 sticks celery
Net carbs: 3

Total daily net carbs: 21.5

Week 2

Sunday

Breakfast
Leftover Keto Biscuits and Gravy, 1 serving
Net carbs: 7

Lunch

Leftover Keto clam chowder: 1 serving
Net carbs: 6

Dinner
Portobello-Stuffed Burger, 1 serving
Net carbs: 4

Snack
Leftover Keto chocolate chip waffles/pancakes: 2 pancakes
Net carbs: 4

Dessert:
Leftover Red Velvet Fat Bombs, 2 servings
Net carbs: 2

Total daily net carbs: 23

Monday

Breakfast
2 hard-boiled eggs with a little melted butter (Cook up 4, because we'll eat the rest on Weds!)
Net carbs: 1

Lunch
Leftover Keto clam chowder: 1 serving
Net carbs: 6

Dinner
Garlic Butter Steak and Caprese
Net carbs: 4.5

Snack
Quesadilla and salsa, 1 serving
Net carbs: 4

Total daily net carbs: 15.5

Tuesday

Breakfast
1 serving of Keto Biscuits and Gravy
Net carbs: 7

Lunch
Leftover Keto clam chowder: 1 serving
Net carbs: 6

Dinner
Low-carb egg rolls, 1 serving
Net carbs: 7

Snack
¼ C. salted almonds
Net carbs: 3

Dessert
Chocolate Mascarpone Mousse, 2 servings (We'll eat the rest later!)
Net carbs: 3

Total daily net carbs: 27 (Make sure you watch your extra carbs today!)

Wednesday

Breakfast
2 hard-boiled eggs with a little melted butter
Net carbs: 1

Lunch
Leftover Keto clam chowder: 1 serving
Net carbs: 6

Dinner
Keto Personal Pepperoni Pizza, 1 serving
Net carbs: 5

Snack
Leftover Low-Carb Egg Rolls, 1 serving
Net carbs: 7

Dessert:
Leftover Red Velvet Fat Bombs, 2 servings
Net carbs: 2

Total daily net carbs 22

Thursday

Breakfast
½ C. yogurt with stevia topped with ¼ C. sliced strawberries
Net carbs: 4.5

Lunch
Leftover Keto clam chowder: 1 serving
Net carbs: 6

Dinner
Artichoke Chicken, 1 serving (Save remaining servings for lunch!)
Net carbs: 4

Snack
Leftover Low-Carb Egg Rolls, 1 serving
Net carbs: 7

Total daily net carbs: 21.5

Friday

Breakfast
1 serving of low-carb chocolate protein shake
Net carbs: 3

Lunch
Leftover Artichoke Chicken, 1 serving (Save the remaining servings for lunch!)
Net carbs: 4

Dinner
Deluxe Keto Burger, 1 serving
Net carbs: 2.5

Snack
Pork rinds, 1 serving
Net carbs: 0

Dessert
Leftover Chocolate Mascarpone Mousse, 2 servings
Net carbs: 3

Total daily net carbs: 12.5

Saturday

Breakfast
Keto chocolate chip waffles/pancakes: 2 pancakes (From your frozen stash!)
Net carbs: 4

Lunch
Leftover Artichoke Chicken, 1 serving (Save the remaining servings for lunch!)
Net carbs: 4

Dinner
Keto Chopped Salad, 1 serving
Net carbs: 6.5

Snack
Pork rinds, 1 serving
Net carbs: 0

Dessert:
Leftover Red Velvet Fat Bombs, 2 servings
Net carbs: 2

Total daily net carbs: 16.5

CHAPTER 15
Cheating on Keto the Smart Way

The very FIRST question that many people ask when they start keto (or think about starting keto) is "how often can I cheat and still get the results I want?"

There's a reason I didn't cover this question first—even though it's typically the first question a lot of people ask. By this point in the book, I hope you understand that when you stick to the keto diet (especially for those first three pivotal weeks), the desire to stuff your face with a bunch of carbs WILL drastically diminish.

This means that while you now can't imagine going a week without full-carb pizza or ice cream, the you three weeks from now isn't going to feel super stressed about it. It might sound good, sure. But it won't be a drug-like craving anymore.

So, the first piece of advice I'm going to give you about cheating is this: Wait at LEAST three weeks before you cheat for the first time. Before that, you haven't given yourself nearly enough time to get the withdrawals out of your system. And even then, I'd really advise you to follow these key pieces of advice when you do cheat. And to be clear, I DO recommend that you cheat. Food is joyful, and it's okay to splurge and enjoy something totally frivolous (nutrient-wise) once in a while. Here are my tips for "cheating" in a way that will allow you to reach your goals:

Set Cheat Goals

We typically think of "cheating" as something that happens on the spur of the moment, or when we just can't go another second without giving in to temptation. But I want you to scrub that idea from your brain. Cheating isn't bad. Cheating doesn't make you a failure. And that's why you don't need to do it in secret or as a result of a weak moment.

Plan how often you'd like to enjoy a different, carby meal. And then look forward to that! I'd recommend once or twice a month as a good, healthy number that allows you to look forward to regular non-keto meals, while helping you stay on track and enjoy the benefits of ketosis most of the time. That brings us nicely to our next point!

Cheat MEALS, not Cheat DAYS

Eating a ton of high-carb food for an entire day while sticking to a keto diet otherwise is going to do two things: It's going to make readjusting back to ketosis a little harder. And it's going to bring back cravings harder. Not to mention, it's going to go a long way to offset all the calories you've been cutting (all while feeling full!) on the keto diet.

For that reason, think about your cheats in terms of meals, not days. Two MEALS a month (or one!) instead of two DAYS a month. I make exceptions to this piece of advice during the holidays. On Thanksgiving, Christmas, and Easter, I do whatever I want for the whole day. And often, that means primarily eating keto. Because that's what my body likes and what I enjoy after becoming fat adapted. But you do you, boo! And if you want to eat like days of yore the whole day long on a couple of special holidays, do it! None of us will live forever, even with the health benefits of keto. So make a plan that will work for you, makes you feel good physically and emotionally, and stick to it.

Make the Cheats Count

Again, the whole point of a cheat meal is to enjoy yourself. That means, we're gonna set some ground rules right now: No guilting yourself, no worrying about calories, and no stressing about whether you've "set yourself back." Cheat meals are meant to be enjoyed. You planned for this. Now you get to enjoy it. And then get right back to keto!

I recommend planning your cheat meals around social gatherings or other dates where you're likely to be sharing food with others or celebrating something. Sometimes it's just nice to eat what everyone else is eating in social situations, and planning (or saving) your cheat meals a couple of times a month for these gatherings can make keto significantly more sustainable.

Plan on a Tough First Cheat

The longer you stick with keto, the easier it is to bounce back after a cheat. But with those first cheats, your body still remembers all too well the easy, tantalizing energy simple carbs offer. That's why those first few cheats can bring up some resurgence in cravings afterward. Prepare for this to happen and make a plan to deal with those cravings the way you did during the first few weeks of adaptation. You've got this, and it only gets easier.

How Many Carbs Will Kick Me Out of Ketosis?

The short answer is, it doesn't take much. Just one bagel or a big banana will do it. So don't tell yourself the cheat meal "doesn't count" if it was "just a bagel." If you think with that mindset, you're going to be cheating a lot more often than you tell yourself. And your results will show it!

Know What to Expect After a Cheat Meal

After a cheat meal, just know you're going to retain some water. That is NOT fat, and it does NOT mean that you've suddenly and immediately gained back a bunch of the weight you've lost. If your pants feel a little tighter the day after, or your scale says you've really blown your goals, don't panic. It's water weight, and it'll go away.

The majority of the carbs you eat during any cheat meal are going to be used to replenish your muscles' glycogen stores—not end up as fat deposits. So don't stress.

You might notice a "sugar rush" if your cheat meal is especially carby, with an accompanying rush of energy. And you might also notice a bit of a crash as your body dips back into using glucose and carbs for fuel, with the accompanying roller coaster.

The ketosis faucet will turn down to a mere trickle while you switch back to glucose temporarily. But as your body senses that the carbs have stopped coming in, that faucet will open back up again, and you'll transition back to keto/back to using fat for fuel. The longer you stick with a keto diet, and the more your body adapts to using fat for fuel, the easier it will be to transition back to fat.

Remember, a Cheat Meal Won't Undo Your Progress

This is especially important to remember if your primary goal is losing weight. The keto diet helps you lose weight through regulating blood sugar and controlling cravings. But at the very simplest level, it allows you to reduce your calorie intake (while feeling full and enjoying yummy foods). A cheat meal here or there isn't going to bump your calorie intake up enough to bridge the deficit you've created through sticking with the diet 98 percent of the time. So again, don't stress. Plan for your cheats, enjoy them, and stick to keto the rest of the time!

Embrace Cheating as Part of a Sustainable Diet

I fully advocate for cheating. Many coaches and keto aficionados don't. And that's okay. The most important thing is for YOU to do what works for your goals, lifestyle, and perspective on life. For me, cheating once or twice a month with a carby meal allows me to sustain keto as a lifestyle without feeling deprived. It also allows me to enjoy social situations and holidays more fully. I typically find that (in diet and elsewhere) a flexible approach tends to work better than a rigid one. But that's just me. I know some friends who fall off the wagon completely every time they enjoy a cheat meal. If that's you, I have some alternative ideas to cheating:

Cheats That Aren't Cheats

Sometimes you'll feel like a cheat meal you haven't planned for. Sometimes you'll find that cheating just derails you and isn't a great idea. In that case, I've found that "faux" cheat meals can be very helpful. Here's how you do it: Figure out what you're craving. Pizza? Tacos? Ice cream? Spaghetti? Then make the keto alternative. There are SO many great and delicious options that can scratch that itch without taking you out of ketosis. (A lot of them are included as recipes in this book for that very reason!)

Most of the time, I find that the desire to cheat disappears after enjoying a keto-friendly substitute for what I've been craving. When I'm full of that tasty food, I don't usually feel amped up for an unexpected cheat meal anymore.

Plan Cheat Meals Around Exercise

If you find yourself with an unplanned cheat meal on your hands (e.g., dinner at your boss's house where it's just not an option to eat keto and still enjoy the meal), planning for exercise in conjunction with your cheat meal can help reduce the impact.

Your body is all about that quick source of energy—and it will naturally use that easy-access glucose to fuel you during a workout. Don't try to game the system by planning carb-fests followed by intense workouts. You'll only make your stomach hurt. But thoughtfully pairing exercise with moderate cheat meals can help offset some of that carbiness by turning it into exercise fuel.

Have the Right Mindset

Sticking to any diet without a margin of flexibility is a setup for failure, in my experience. You're a person, not a machine. And being thoughtful about cheat meals can actually help amplify the effects of keto in reaching your goals, if they allow you to stick with the diet more sustainably. Cheat meals can also help you stay motivated and mark your progress as you stick with your new way of eating.

Keto only works if you stick with it. And cheat meals help me do just that: stick with it. Remember though, YOU get to decide what works best for you. Take ownership of your keto experience and find what helps you stay motivated while reaching your goals.

CHAPTER 16
Keto and Exercise

One of the top "critiques" and questions I hear about the keto diet is, "How can you expect me to exercise without carb-loading?"

The short answer is that a lot of top athletes (and those man-bros I mentioned in the introduction) use keto as an edge on the competition for athletic performance. Because SO many studies link the keto diet with improved performance.

I felt like a short chapter on keto and exercise was important to set aside some myths and misconceptions about keto and exercise. And to explain why keto and exercise work together so well!

Metabolic Flexibility for the Win

Let's start with WHY keto is great for exercise. Remember that metabolic flexibility we've talked about throughout the book? That comes in exceptionally useful while exercising. Because when your body adapts to using fat and ketones for fuel, it can more easily tap into stored fat as well as consumed calories during exercise.

That means less fatigue, better endurance, and improved fat loss (win, win, win).

Exercise Can Help with Carb Withdrawals

Look, I get it. When you're craving a pizza and donuts and deep in the throes of carb withdrawal, the last thing you want to do is go for a light jog or a hike. But the thing is, exercise can actually speed up the transition to fat adaption, since it forces your body to get creative with energy and stabilize your blood sugar in order to function. And that means fewer carb cravings!

Keto + Exercise to Reach Goals Faster

Whether your keto goals include more mental clarity, reducing inflammation, improving your endurance, or losing weight, exercise can help you reach your goals more efficiently with keto.

Here are a few key tips for using exercise effectively while on keto:

1. **Be conscientious about refueling electrolytes.** Remember, keto ALREADY taps into your electrolytes (potassium, magnesium, and calcium) more heavily. When you add sweat and exercise to the equation, you really need to be diligent about refueling. Failing to do so can result in muscle cramps, difficulty sleeping, and fatigue.

2. **Get enough calories.** Like I keep telling you, the goal of the keto diet is NOT to white-knuckle your way through an exercise in starvation. Your goal is to get more in tune with your body's signals for real hunger by eliminating refined carbs and moderating complex carbs. You need fuel. Especially when you're exercising. So make sure you're eating when your body tells you that you're hungry, while aligning your food choices with your daily macros.

3. **Add a few extra carbs after heavy workouts.** If you're running marathons (or preparing to do so), you're going to need a few extra carbs beyond what I've outlined in this book. Consuming the bulk of your daily carbs in small pre- and post-workout meals can help you with muscle recovery and insulin sensitivity.

Maximizing Different Kinds of Exercise with Keto

Regardless of your preferred type of exercise, you'll find it's a good pair with keto. The follow are some of the most popular forms of exercise and a few tips:

Strength Training

One of the myths about carbs is that it's impossible to build muscle without them. I'm happy to report that's not true. If you're getting enough protein, you'll find that strength training and muscle building can be incredibly effective with keto.

If you're doing an intensive strength-training regimen, pay special attention to your protein intake. You can also try supplementing with creatine to improve your results.

HIIT Workouts

HIIT workouts (high-intensity interval training) have gotten really popular. It's where you wear yourself out in short bursts. This helps keep your body on its toes, so to speak, instead of finding equilibrium with a sustained exercise pace. For that reason, HIIT workouts can use a lot of calories and fuel weight loss.

Just remember to fuel your body. You can't run on empty and expect great results. You'll want to keep your HIIT workouts to around 3 times per week.

Aerobic Exercise

Steady exercise that gets the heart pumping is a fantastic match with the keto diet, since your body now has the ability to tap into fat stores more easily and improve your endurance. Just remember to watch your electrolytes and protein intake, so you stay fueled up!

So Many Exercise Goodies

This chapter is really just scratching the surface when it comes to the benefits of exercise and keto. Exercise also improves insulin sensitivity, mood, cardiovascular health, and stress levels. Basically, I highly recommend incorporating exercise into your keto diet regardless of your goals.

This isn't an exercise book. But I can vouch for the idea that incorporating exercise into your lifestyle is a great way to fully embrace a healthier lifestyle rather than a temporary stint with surface-level changes. And that's essential for lasting and meaningful change!

CHAPTER 17
What You Need to Know About Intermittent Fasting and Keto

This isn't a book about fasting. That topic deserves its own book. And if you want to read one of those, I highly recommend *The Obesity Code* by Jason Fung.

That said, the topics of keto and intermittent fasting come up together over and over again. So let's talk about why:

Why Keto and Fasting?

Combining keto with fasting (like combining keto with exercise) can be incredibly powerful (but don't combine the three for long periods of time, because again: you need fuel).

Fasting all by itself is actually pretty darn cool. There's a TON of research (and a Nobel Prize recently awarded) that shows benefits like disease prevention, extended lifespan, and a boost to the immune system (to name just a few).

The great thing about keto is that it removes one of the biggest hurdles to fasting: adaptation to using fat for fuel. Most people who dive straight into a fasted state deal with irritability and carb withdrawals. But you've already done that. Which means you can skip straight to the benefits and more easily transition into a fully fasted state. Most people require a fast of one or two days to start seeing benefits of a fast. If you're on a keto, a fast of as little as 14 hours can yield those benefits (and yes, some of those hours can be sleeping hours!)

We'll talk about the guidelines of a successful fast in just a second. First, let's talk about the benefits of fasting. Because I know a lot of you are thinking, "You want me to go hungry WHY? I thought we weren't doing that." And the answer is yes, I'm a big advocate for not going hungry. Fasting is the one exception, and I'm telling you right now that you DON'T have to do it. You can very much succeed at keto without it. But I'm telling you, you might decide to try it (like many keto dieters) after learning about some of the cool benefits.

Benefits of Fasting

Remember that Nobel Peace Prize I told you about? It was awarded to the person who discovered WHY fasting yields so many health benefits. Scientists have known for a long time that fasting does indeed improve health. But they had no real idea of why.

And then someone finally pinpointed something called "autophagy." Autophagy is a unique state the body enters during fasting, in which old, diseased, and damaged cells are consumed and recycled as fuel. T-cells get activated, and the body essentially goes into "deep cleaning" mode. Our ancestors entered autophagy regularly. Because food wasn't stocked on shelves and in grocery stores. Spending a couple of days without much food was a normal thing, and the body learned to take advantage of this circumstance. But in modern society, many of us don't miss even a single meal. Here's a few of the top benefits of fasting and autophagy:

Cellular Repair and Removal of Waste Buildup

Autophagy is like spring cleaning for your body on a cellular level. During a fasted state, your body will cannibalize damaged cells, recycle and clean up waste, and go into a heightened state of repair and renewal.

Lowered Inflammation and Oxidative Stress

Fasting has been shown to lower inflammation and stress on the cells and organs. This is especially true for keto dieters, since sugar is tightly linked with inflammation. Many people with inflammatory diseases like arthritis, Crohn's, and psoriasis notice significant improvement with regular fasting.

Better Mental Health

Incredibly, some studies have found that fasting is as powerful as antidepressants. There's some debate over why this happens, but most experts believe this has something to do with the fact that fasting (and keto!) stabilize blood sugar and reduce inflammation in all areas of the body, including the brain.

A Fast Track to Ketosis

A short fast can speed up the amount of time it takes to really turn on the faucet of ketosis. Some people follow a cheat meal with a short fast to help turn that faucet back on more quickly.

Longer Life

I know this sounds crazy, but there's a lot of evidence to show that regular fasting can improve lifespan by as much as 30 percent. This is the likely result of ALL the different benefits of fasting (better cellular health, immune strength, reduced inflammation, etc.)

Better Immune Response

During a fast, your "killer-T" cells (the backbone of your immune response) kick into high gear. They aggressively seek out damaged cells, immune threats, and infection. This can help address budding disease threats (like precancerous cells and pathogens). In several animal studies, fasting helps speed up recovery from bacterial infections.

The Basics of a Successful Fast

Like keto, you need to understand a few things about fasting BEFORE you jump right in, for a good experience and to reap the most rewards.

On the one hand, fasting is as simple as abstaining from food/caloric intake for a set amount of time. However, to get the most benefits (and even enjoy) a fast, keep the following best practices in mind:

1. **Decide how long you want to fast**. I recommend starting slow, with a short fast to gain confidence. Try a 16-hour

fast first, then a 24-hour fast, and then a 3-5 day fast (if you want). You don't have to fast as part of the keto diet, but if it's something you want to try, ease yourself into it! There's no race. If you're going to fast longer than 3-5 days, make sure you talk to a doctor first (and be very mindful of the remaining tips).

2. **Decide how often you want to fast.** Some people choose to fast 14-16 hours every single day. Others choose to fast 24-hours once a week. Still others decide to fast once a month. How often you fast will depend on your health goals, how you feel while fasting, and your lifestyle.

3. **Listen to your body.** Fasting is a great way to really get in tune with your body. A few hunger pangs are normal (and will pass), but nausea, strong headaches, or hunger pains that deepen and last, that's your body telling you to stop. Listen to it and break your fast.

4. **The longer the fast, the slower you refuel after.** For longer fasts, you're going to want to refuel slowly afterward (instead of planning a big meal). Eating a ton of calories all at once can really disrupt your electrolyte balance and make you feel awful. In some cases, it can even be very dangerous (and is called "refeeding syndrome.") The longer the fast, the more important it is for you to refuel slowly and carefully. E.g., start with some broth.

5. **Keep electrolytes balanced.** Keto acts like a diuretic already. And so does fasting. You'll need to stay hydrated and keep your electrolyte levels high. Some people choose to supplement with electrolytes like magnesium, potassium, and calcium during a fast. This will help stave off headaches, nausea, and fatigue.

6. **Remember, the goal isn't going hungry.** The goal is adopting a new tool that can benefit your overall health. Fasting isn't about starvation, willpower, or even weight loss. It's an opportunity to connect with your body in a new way and improve your overall health.

I know fasting sounds weird at first (just like keto!), but I'd encourage you to do your own research. There are literally thousands of peer-reviewed, large-scale, longitudinal studies that show incredible benefits. Basically, don't take my word for it. I'm not a doctor. I'm your well-informed friend. But I've done a WHOLE lot of research, and I'd encourage you to verify what I'm telling you (as with everything else in this book or any other).

Who SHOULDN'T Fast?

If you are pregnant, have trouble making your own insulin (e.g., you have diabetes), or your kidneys or liver are compromised (e.g., you have hepatitis or kidney disease), you'll want to talk to a doctor before you fast.

Short fasts are safe for most people (I mean, most of us go around 10 hours without eating at night. Adding a few more hours is pretty darn doable!). But if you have any questions or aren't sure, talk to your doctor!

CHAPTER 18
Pep Talk: Do NOT Read Until You Need It

You're reading it anyway, aren't you?

Rebel.

Kidding. But in all seriousness, I want to remind you of two things if you're feeling like giving up (or if you fell off the bandwagon and are knee-deep in a pile of carbs).

First, the keto diet isn't about perfection. It's about finding a tool that can help you reach your goals and feel healthier. You don't have to do it perfectly to benefit. And you don't have to feel bad if you decide to take a break or get side-tracked.

Second, are you enjoying your meals and your experience with keto? If not, why? Can that be changed? Because white-knuckling your way through any diet or lifestyle is a recipe for burnout and stress and despair. The journey is always going to feel like the destination. And if you're not enjoying this keto journey, it's time to find a way to tweak that experience. Take a look at your perspective. Are you expecting perfection and feeling upset when you fall short? Knock that off right now. You're just fine the way you are. And this is just a tool. Are you enjoying the food you're eating on a daily basis? If not, it's time to find new go-to meals you really enjoy. Are you feeling deprived of some of your old favorites? Maybe it's time to find some yummy substitutes—or enjoy some more cheat meals.

You can do this. Don't worry about a month from now or a year from now too much. Focus on the next little thing, then do it. And then the next. You've got this.

A Note From the Author

If you enjoyed this book, a positive review would mean the world to me. Like other small-press authors, I rely heavily on word-of-mouth recommendations to reach new readers.

I can promise you that I read every single review. Because if you enjoyed this book or it helped you, you're the one I wrote it for!

Made in United States
North Haven, CT
17 May 2024

52655616R10085